T0250022

Digitalization and Innovation in Health

Providing a comparison between context in Europe and the US, this volume investigates the digital transformation of health systems, comparing strategies for digital development while identifying both key innovations and future challenges.

The book covers a wide spectrum of topics, from explaining the nature of individual innovations to an analysis of demand-side and supply-side barriers, including funding issues and technological access. It also explores where digitalization is already playing an important role, for example, in clinical trials and disease modeling.

Concluding with guidance for policy recommendations, this important book will interest students, scholars, and practitioners across health and social care, medicine, and beyond.

Marzenna Anna Weresa is Professor at the SGH Warsaw School of Economics, Poland; director of the World Economy Research Institute, Poland; a member of the Microeconomics of Competitiveness Affiliate Network at Harvard Business School, Boston; a principal investigator in research projects financed by FP7, Horizon 2020, Bloomberg Initiative Grants, and COST Actions; and an expert for the European Commission on policies for research and innovation. Her research focuses on innovation systems and policy, digital transformation, FDI, international trade, and competitiveness.

Christina Ciecierski is a Professor in the Department of Economics, co-director of the Center of Health and principal investigator for the Chicago Cancer Health Equity Collaborative (Chicago CHEC) at Northeastern Illinois University, US. Her research focuses on consumer health behaviors, health disparities, and policy. Research reported in this publication is supported, in part, by the National Institutes of Health's National Cancer Institute, Grant Numbers U54CA202995, U54CA202997, and U54CA203000. The content is solely the responsibility of the authors and does not necessarily represent the official views of the National Institutes of Health.

Lidia Filus is Professor and chair of Mathematics, Northeastern Illinois University, US, and principal investigator at Chicago Cancer Health Equity Collaborative (ChicagoCHEC), Northeastern Illinois University, US. Research reported in this publication is supported, in part, by the National Institutes of Health's National Cancer Institute, Grant Numbers U54CA202995, U54CA202997, and U54CA203000. The content is solely the responsibility of the authors and does not necessarily represent the official views of the National Institutes of Health.

Digitalization and Innovation in Health

European and US Perspectives

Edited by
Marzenna Anna Weresa,
Christina Ciecierski
and Lidia Filus

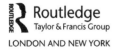

Routledge
Taylor & Francis Group

LONDON AND NEW YORK

First published 2024
by Routledge
4 Park Square, Milton Park, Abingdon, Oxon OX14 4RN

and by Routledge
605 Third Avenue, New York, NY 10158

Routledge is an imprint of the Taylor & Francis Group, an informa business

British Library Cataloguing-in-Publication Data
A catalogue record for this book is available from the British Library

Library of Congress Cataloging-in-Publication Data
Names: Weresa, Marzenna A., editor. | Filus, Lidia, editor. | Ciecierski,
Christina, editor.
Title: Digitalization and innovation in health: European and US
perspectives / edited by Marzenna Anna Weresa, Christina Ciecierski
and Lidia Filus.
Description: Abingdon, Oxon; New York, NY: Routledge, 2024. |
Includes bibliographical references and index. |
Identifiers: LCCN 2024000086 (print) | LCCN 2024000087 (ebook) |
ISBN 9781032726496 (hbk) | ISBN 9781032726519 (pbk) |
ISBN 9781032726557 (ebk)
Classification: LCC R858 .D5445 2024 (print) | LCC R858 (ebook) |
DDC 610.285—dc23/eng/20240118
LC record available at https://lccn.loc.gov/2024000086
LC ebook record available at https://lccn.loc.gov/2024000087

ISBN: 978-1-032-72649-6 (hbk)
ISBN: 978-1-032-72651-9 (pbk)
ISBN: 978-1-032-72655-7 (ebk)

DOI: 10.4324/9781032726557

Typeset in Times New Roman
by codeMantra

Contents

List of figures		*vii*
List of tables		*xi*
List of contributors		*xiii*
Acknowledgments		*xvii*

Introduction 1
MARZENNA ANNA WERESA, CHRISTINA CIECIERSKI AND
LIDIA FILUS

PART 1
Digital Innovation in Health: Setting the Scene 5

**1 Nature of Digital Health Innovation: Mapping
the Research Field** 7
MARZENNA ANNA WERESA
AND SCOTT WILLIAM HEGERTY

**2 Digital Readiness in Healthcare: Comparative Analysis
of EU and US Resources and Capabilities** 18
ARKADIUSZ MICHAŁ KOWALSKI,
MAŁGORZATA STEFANIA LEWANDOWSKA
AND DAWID MAJCHEREK

**3 Funding of the Digital Health Transformation
in the US: Comparative Study of Venture Capital
and Initial Public Offering** 35
IZABELA PRUCHNICKA-GRABIAS

PART 2
Digitalization of Health Systems: Evidence from Poland   61

4 **Digital Health Index in Poland: A Comparative Perspective**   63
JULIAN SMÓŁKA AND MARTYNA SMÓŁKA

5 **Teleconsultations in Poland: Will the COVID-driven
Popularization of Teleconsultations Turn into
a Long-Lasting Strategy?**   85
BARBARA WIĘCKOWSKA, MONIKA RAULINAJTYS-GRZYBEK
AND KATARZYNA BYSZEK

PART 3
Digitalization in Medical Research Practice   111

6 **Adaptation of Time Series Analysis to Central
Statistical Monitoring of Clinical Trials: A Pilot Study**   113
MACIEJ FRONC

7 **Generalized Diffusion Model to Understand
and Predict Viral Spread**   132
PAULO H. ACIOLI

Conclusions and Implications   148
MARZENNA ANNA WERESA, CHRISTINA CIECIERSKI
AND LIDIA FILUS

Index   153

Figures

1.1 Number of papers on digital health innovations in the
    Web of Science database by year of publication
    in 2014–2023   10
1.2 Distribution of citations per year   10
1.3 The most important research themes centered
    around digital health innovations: the analysis of the
    co-occurrence of keywords in publications indexed
    in the WoS database in 2014–2023 (n=142)   13
2.1 Countries in terms of healthy life expectancy (in years)
    and domestic general government health expenditure
    (% of GDP)   25
2.2 Countries in terms of healthy life expectancy (in years)
    and number of physicians (per 1,000 people)   27
2.3 Countries according to percentage of the population
    using the Internet to seek health information and
    domestic private healthcare expenditure as a percentage
    of current healthcare expenditure   27
2.4 Countries in terms of percentage of the population using
    the Internet to seek health information and general
    Internet usage   28
3.1 Directions and stages of capital flow in a venture
    capital process   38
3.2 Stock market quotations for the S&P Kensho index from
    January 1, 2014 to May 11, 2023 (USD)   43
3.3 Stock market quotations of the S&P500 Total Return
    index from January 1, 2014 to May 11, 2023 (USD)   45
3.4 Daily prices of Bitcoin from January 1, 2014 to May 11,
    2023 (USD)   45
3.5 Daily prices of Brent crude oil from January 1,
    2014 to May 11, 2023 (USD)   46
4.1 Digital health maturity overview for Poland: proxy data,
    study results   80
5.1 Share of teleconsultations in the total number of GP
    services by month (September 2020–December 2021)   91

5.2 Share of teleconsultations in the total number
of GP services by voivodeship (2021)   92

5.3 Share of teleconsultations in the total number of AOS
services by month (2020–2021)   94

5.4 Share of teleconsultations in the total number of AOS
services by voivodeship (2021)   94

5.5 Share of teleservices in the total number of psychiatric
care services for adults by voivodeship (2021)   97

5.6 Share of teleconsultations in the total number of
long-term care services by type and month (2021)   100

6.1 Correlation heatmap for selected variables   119

6.2 Variability over time supplemented with ACF and PACF
plots for CACRALB, subject 2   120

6.3 Forecast comparison for CACRALB, subject 2   122

6.4 Outlier detection for CACRALB, subject 2   124

6.5 Variability over time supplemented with ACF and PACF
plots for LYM, subject 192   125

6.6 Forecast comparison for LYM, subject 192   127

6.7 Outlier detection for LYM, subject 192   128

7.1 The number of infected individuals (full line) in a
logarithmic scale and the exponential fit for the initial
ten days of the simulation (dashed line) averaged over
50–90-day simulations of the spread of a virus in a
population of 100 individuals in a square cell with the
population density of the city of (a) NYC (0.0120 people/
m^2) (b) Chicago (0.0047 people/m^2). D =100 m^2/day,
prob = 0.2, dt = 0.01 day, r_{transm} = 1 m.   135

7.2 The number of infected individuals in a logarithmic
scale as a function of the diffusion constant averaged
over 20 90-day simulations of the spread of a virus
in a population of 1,000 individuals in a square cell
with the population density of the city of (a) NYC
($\rho = 0.012$ people/m^2) (b) Chicago ($\rho = 0.0047$ people/m^2).
$D = 100$ m^2/day, prob = 0.1, dt = 0.01 day, r_{transm} = 2 m   136

7.3 Snapshots of a single simulation of 10,000 people
arranged in a simulation cell with the density of the
city of Chicago. The color-coded spheres correspond to
healthy (grey), infected (black), and recovered
(light grey) individuals   138

7.4 Example of a two-diffusion constant simulation cell with
1,000 individuals. The left side of the cell has a diffusion
constant D_1 and the right has a diffusion constant D_2. The
initial population is uniformly distributed over the whole
simulation cell   139

7.5   Population density as a function of time for a
        two-diffusion constant simulation cell with initial
        population density of 0.0047 people/m^2. The black
        line represents the high diffusion constant side
        (D_1 = 106.4 m^2/day). The grey line represents the low
        diffusion constant side (D_2 = 41.7 m^2/day)   139
7.6   Population density as a function of time for a
        two-diffusion constant simulation cell with initial
        population density of 0.00835 people/m^2. The black line
        represents the high diffusion constant side (D_1 = 106.4
        m^2/day). The grey line represents the low diffusion
        constant side (D_2 = 41.7 m^2/day)   140
7.7   Comparison of the number of cases of two towns
        (Towns 1 and 2) with fixed diffusion constants with
        a two-diffusion constant simulation cell with initial
        population density. The black line represents Town 1
        (D_1 = 106.4 m^2/day). The dark grey line represents Town 2
        (D_2 = 41.7 m^2/day). The light grey line represents Town 3
        (ρ_3 = 0.00835 people/m^2, D_1 = 106.4 m^2/day, D_2 = 41.7 m^2/day)   141
7.8   Number of cases (in logarithmic scale) as a function of
        time for a simulation of two interacting 1,000 people
        towns with the population densities of Chicago (Town 1)
        and NYS (Town 2). The first contaminated individual
        was in Town 1   142
7.9   Number of cases (in logarithmic scale) as a function of
        time for a simulation of two interacting 1,000 people
        towns with the population densities of Chicago (Town 1)
        and NYS (Town 2). The first contaminated individual
        was in Town 2   142
7.10   Comparison of the number of cases (in logarithmic scale)
        as a function of time for a simulation of 100 population
        towns for different social distance levels of compliance.
        The lines represent different compliance levels: No
        compliance (black), 25% compliance (dark grey), 50%
        compliance (grey), and 75% compliance (light grey).The
        top panel represents a tow with the population density of
        Chicago. The bottom panel represents a town with the
        population density of NYC   145

Tables

1.1	Data selection process	8
1.2	Journals with multiple appearances in each group	11
1.3	Common keywords by group	12
1.4	Countries with the highest proportions of author affiliations	12
1.5	Definitions of digital innovation in health	14
2.1	Summary statistics of data related to digital readiness and macroeconomic determinants	23
2.2	Final recommendations for further healthcare digitalization in different regions	29
S1	Database	33
3.1	Venture capital invested in digital health in 2011–2023	40
3.2	Correlation table for analyzed assets	47
3.3	Descriptive statistics of logarithmic returns on the S&P500 TR Index from January 1, 2014 to May 11, 2023	48
3.4	Descriptive statistics of logarithmic returns on the S&P500 TR Kensho Index from January 1, 2014 to May 11, 2023	49
3.5	Descriptive statistics of logarithmic returns on Bitcoin from January 1, 2014 to May 1, 2023	50
3.6	Descriptive statistics of logarithmic returns on Brent crude oil from January 1, 2014 to May 11, 2023	50
3.7	Main statistics of logarithmic returns on the S&P500 TR Index from January 1, 2014 to May 11, 2023 divided into subperiods	51
3.8	Main statistics of logarithmic returns on the S&P Kensho TR Index from January 1, 2014 to May 11, 2023 divided into subperiods	52
3.9	Main statistics of logarithmic returns on Bitcoin from January 1, 2014 to May 11, 2023 divided into subperiods	54
3.10	Main statistics of logarithmic returns on crude oil from January 1, 2014 to May 11, 2023 divided into subperiods	55

4.1 Selected digital health maturity assessment models comparison — 65
4.2 Results summary concerning Leadership & Governance category in Polish digital health — 69
4.3 Results summary in the area concerning Strategy & Investment category in Polish digital health — 71
4.4 Results summary concerning Legislation, Policy, & Compliance category in Polish digital health — 73
4.5 Results summary concerning the Workforce category in Polish digital health — 74
4.6 Results summary concerning Standards & Interoperability category in Polish digital health — 75
4.7 Results summary concerning Infrastructure category in Polish digital health — 76
4.8 Results summary concerning Services & Applications category in Polish digital health — 78
5.1 Share of teleconsultations in the total number of GP services by age groups (2020–2021) — 92
5.2 Structure of services in psychiatric care services for adults (2021) — 96
5.3 Structure of services in psychiatric care services for youth and children (2021) — 97
5.4 Structure of services in palliative and hospice care (2021) — 101
6.1 Laboratory variables involved in the analysis — 116
6.2 ADF test results for CACRALB, subject 2 — 121
6.3 ETS model summary for CACRALB, subject 2 — 121
6.4 ARIMA model summary for CACRALB, subject 2 — 121
6.5 Forecast accuracy for CACRALB, subject 2 — 121
6.6 ADF test results for LYM, subject 192 — 126
6.7 ETS model summary for LYM, subject 192 — 126
6.8 ARIMA model summary for LYM, subject 192 — 126
6.9 Forecast summary for LYM, subject 192 — 126
7.1 Exponential growth rate as a function of diffusion constant for obtained from the first ten days of simulation of 1,000 individuals in cities with densities corresponding to New York City and Chicago — 137
7.2 Exponential growth rate as a function of diffusion constant for obtained from the first 10 days of simulation of 1,000 individuals with one random traveler per day in each city — 138

Contributors

Paulo H. Acioli works in the Department of Physics and Astronomy at Northeastern Illinois University, US. Dr Acioli is a Professor of physics and contributing to computational modeling in physical chemistry, sustainable energy, education in STEM, spiral waves, population interactions, and viral diffusion spread. His research interests are modeling the use of mixed-metal clusters in single-atom catalysis, use of cellular automata to study multi-species predator-prey interactions, diffusion modeling of viral spread, and STEM education.

Katarzyna Byszek holds a PhD degree from the Collegium of Socio-Economics at the SGH Warsaw School of Economics, Poland. She examines the impact of regulations on cross-border healthcare and finances new technologies in the health industry.

Maciej Fronc is a graduate of the SGH Warsaw School of Economics in quantitative methods in economics and information systems and of Warsaw University of Technology in biotechnology and chemical and process engineering. He is a PhD student in management and quality studies. Since 2021, he has been working for GSK as a central statistical monitor. His research focuses on the implementation of quantitative methods in the pharmaceutical industry for the improvement of the drug development process in the spirit of the quality management theory.

Scott W. Hegerty is Professor of economics and Chair of the Departments of Anthropology, Economics, Geography & Environmental Studies, Global Studies, and Philosophy at Northeastern Illinois University in Chicago, US. He conducts applied statistical research in macroeconomics and urban economics. He received his PhD from the University of Wisconsin-Milwaukee, US.

Arkadiusz Michał Kowalski is Associate Professor in the Collegium of World Economy at the SGH Warsaw School of Economics, Poland. His research and academic teaching focus on innovation policy, clusters, and international competitiveness. He has been involved as a manager or researcher in various European or domestic research projects in these fields, which resulted in more than 100 publications, including books, chapters, articles in scientific journals, and expert reports. He does consultancy work with international organizations, governmental bodies, enterprises, and clusters.

Małgorzata Stefania Lewandowska is Associate Professor in the Department of International Management at the SGH Warsaw School of Economics, Poland; author and co-author of books, papers, and chapters on management in international business, international cooperation of enterprises, business models of firms, and innovation policy. The areas of research are innovation determinants and strategies, open innovation, innovation policy, and eco-innovation. Professor Lewandowska is a member of international associations such as the Academy of International Business (AIB) and the European International Business Academy (EIBA).

Dawid Majcherek is Assistant Professor in the Department of International Management at the SGH Warsaw School of Economics, Poland. He specializes in health economics, sports economics, econometrics, machine learning, clustering, and spatial analysis. He has been working in the pharmaceutical industry since 2013 on various topics related to marketing, sales, management, salesforce effectiveness, finance, and market access including pricing and pharmacoeconomics.

Izabela Pruchnicka-Grabias is an Associate Professor at the SGH Warsaw School of Economics and the Head of the Investment Banking Department. Her research focuses on alternative investments, financial derivatives, finance, and portfolio management. She is the author of about 200 scientific publications. She is an expert for the Warsaw District Court, Wrocław District Court, European Commission, Chancellery of the President of the Republic of Poland, and Bureau of Research at the Sejm of the Republic of Poland.

Monika Raulinajtys-Grzybek is Professor and head of the Department of Managerial Accounting at the SGH Warsaw School of Economics, Poland. Her areas of expertise cover health technology assessment, non-financial reporting and the concept of a business model, management in healthcare, management accounting in healthcare organizations, and pricing of healthcare services.

Julian Smółka studied at the SGH Warsaw School of Economics, Poland; Bocconi University in Milan; and the National University of Singapore. He is a strategy analyst at TUiR Warta, President of the European Foundation for Entrepreneurship Development, and managing director at Dr Smółka Medical Centre.

Martyna Smółka studied at the SGH Warsaw School of Economics, Poland; Bocconi University in Milan; and George Mason University in Washington, DC. She is professionally involved in the finance sector and economic analysis. She gained her professional experience at the KGHM Analytics Centre and Mercatus Center and elsewhere.

Barbara Więckowska is Professor in the Healthcare Innovation Unit at the SGH Warsaw School of Economics, Poland; expert for the Polish Ministry of Health; and co-chair of the DRG change management group in the National Healthcare Fund. She examines financing mechanisms in the healthcare system in Poland. Her research generally focuses on assessing efficiency in healthcare resource allocation.

Acknowledgments

This monograph has been supported by the Polish National Agency for Academic Exchange under the Strategic Partnerships programme, grant number BPI/PST/2021/1/00069/U/00001.

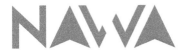

Introduction

Marzenna Anna Weresa,
Christina Ciecierski and Lidia Filus

This book aims to study various dimensions of digital transformation within the health sectors of selected European Union (EU) countries and the United States (US). The emergence of the digital economy, the introduction of Industry 4.0 solutions, climate change, and challenges related to aging societies have led to growing interest in digital innovation among scholars and policymakers. At the same time, due to external shocks such as those created by the COVID-19 pandemic, health-related issues and concerns have emerged as one of the most critical research domains worldwide.

The importance and significance of health and well-being are also reflected in the United Nations Agenda 2030 (UN, 2015) and its social development goals (SDGs), which aim to improve health conditions and well-being for all ages. Growing interests in health coupled with a drive to go digital make the digital health topic interesting and important not only for scholars but also for entire societies. The Covid-19 pandemic initiated a digital health decade and with this, increased the need for digital transformations in health. Digital innovative solutions can improve linkages between patients and healthcare providers, through user application and through digital technological solutions developed for treatment. Digitalization allows for new approaches to medical prevention, health monitoring, and clinical treatment, which may increase efficiency across health sectors (Visconti & Morea, 2020).

Digital transformation, including the implementation of digital innovations and new business models, has been studied across a variety of sectors (e.g., Wade, 2015; OECD, 2021; Kraus et al., 2021; Caputo et al., 2021); however, research on the digitalization of health continues to be fragmented. Some studies focus on selected countries (e.g., the case of Germany by Walzer, 2022) while others focus on individual digital solutions in healthcare (e.g., online treatment by Taylor et al., 2022; Prescot, 2022) or digital innovation (e.g., Roethe et al., 2020; Chelberg et al., 2022; Di Giacomo et al., 2021; Cannavacciuolo et al., 2022).

This book brings together studies that examine a variety of aspects related to the digitalization of the health sector in the European Union (EU) and the US. The analyses presented within relate to both the US and EU Member

DOI: 10.4324/9781032726557-1

States, with Poland taken as a case study for discussing selected aspects of healthcare digitalization. In particular, this book seeks to:

- Map research regarding digital innovation and identify different types of digital innovative solutions (e.g., telemedicine, artificial intelligence, 3-D printing) that contribute to digital transformations in health industries.
- Compare readiness to use digital technologies in accessing healthcare services in the EU and the US.
- Examine funding models of digital health solutions in the US.
- Provide empirical evidence for the implementation of digital health innovations occurring in Poland (case study).
- Present examples of how digital solutions are used in medical research practice.

The book is divided into three parts of which the first focuses on a wide spectrum of digital health topics beginning with an explanation of the nature of digital health innovation, followed by the analysis of digital readiness in healthcare and presentation of financing models. Part two provides a case study of digitalization in health systems while Part three presents specific topics related to the use of big data when analyzing clinical trials and when modeling virus spread.

The novelty of this book is its empirical layer which shows the nature of digital health innovations and how they are applied in health systems in the US and the EU. Study results presented are interdisciplinary in nature and combine economics, finance, and medicine. Through the integration of various disciplines, this book attempts to offer holistic insight into the digitalization of the health sector by incorporating a variety of topics and issues ranging from the use of digital technologies for healthcare delivery (e.g., big data, blockchain, Internet of Things, artificial intelligence) to diagnostics and treatment and finally, big data employment in medical research.

References

Cannavacciuolo, L., Capaldo, G., & Ponsiglione, C. (2022). Digital innovation and organizational changes in the healthcare sector: Multiple case studies of telemedicine project implementation. *Technovation*. https://doi.org/10.1016/j.technovation.2022.102550

Caputo, A., Pizzi, S., Pellegrini, M. M., & Dabić, M. (2021). Digitalization and business models: Where are we going? A science map of the field. *Journal of Business Research, 123*, 489–501.

Chelberg, G. R., Neuhaus, M., Mothershaw, A., Mahoney, R., & Caffery, L. J. (2022). Mobile apps for dementia awareness, support, and prevention – Review and evaluation. *Disability and Rehabilitation, 44*(17), 4909–4920. https://doi.org/10.1080/09638288.2021.1914755

Di Giacomo, D., Guerra, F., Cannita, K., Di Profio, A., & Ranieri, J. (2021). Digital innovation in oncological primary treatment for well-being of patients: Psychological caring as prompt for enhancing quality of life. *Current Oncology, 28*(4), 2452–2465. https://doi.org/10.3390/curroncol28040224

Kraus, S., Jones, P., Kailer, N., Weinmann, A., Chaparro-Banegas, N., & Roig-Tierno, N. (2021). Digital transformation: An overview of the current state of the art of research. *SAGE Open*, 1–15. https://doi.org/10.1177/21582440211047576

OECD. (2021). *The Digital Transformation of SMEs, OECD Studies on SMEs and Entrepreneurship*. OECD Publishing, Paris. https://doi.org/10.1787/bdb9256a-en

Prescot, J. (2022). Online counselling and therapy. *Mental Health and Social Inclusion, 26*(3), 197–2000. https://doi.org/10.1108/MHSI-04-2022-0029

Roethe, A. L., Landgraf, P., Schröder, T., Misch, M., Vajkoczy, P., & Picht, T. (2020). Monitor-based exoscopic 3D4k neurosurgical interventions: A two-phase prospective-randomized clinical evaluation of a novel hybrid device. *Acta Neurochirurgica, 162*, 2949–2961.

Taylor, L., Giles, S., Howitt, S., Ryan, Z., Brooks, E., Radley, L., Thomson, A., Whitaker, E., Knight, F., Hill, C., Violato, M., Waite, P., Raymont, V., Yu, L.-M., Harris, V., Williams, N., & Creswell, C. (2022). A randomised controlled trial to compare clinical and cost-effectiveness of an online parent-led treatment for child anxiety problems with usual care in the context of COVID-19 delivered in Child and Adolescent Mental Health Services in the UK (Co-CAT): A study protocol for a randomised controlled trial. *Trials, 23*, 942. https://doi.org/10.1186/s13063-022-06833-5

UN. (2015). *Transforming Our World: The 2030 Agenda for Sustainable Development*. United Nations, Geneva. https://sdgs.un.org/2030agenda

Visconti, R. M., & Morea, D. (2020). Healthcare digitalization and pay-for-performance incentives in smart hospital project financing. *International Journal of Environmental Research and Public Health, 17*(7), 2318. https://doi.org/10.3390/ijerph17072318

Wade, M. (2015). *Digital Business Transformation. A Conceptual Framework*. Global Center for Digital Business Transformation, Lausanne. https://www.imd.org/contentassets/d0a4d992d38a41ff85de509156475caa/framework

Walzer, S. (Ed.) (2022). *Digital Healthcare in Germany*. Springer International Publishing, Cham. https://doi.org/10.1007/978-3-030-94025-6

Part 1

Digital Innovation in Health

Setting the Scene

1 Nature of Digital Health Innovation

Mapping the Research Field

Marzenna Anna Weresa
and Scott William Hegerty

Introduction

The COVID-19 crisis demonstrated the importance of digital innovation in meeting current and future health challenges. The pandemic caused an abrupt transition to remote healthcare delivery and fostered the introduction of digital innovative solutions for disease monitoring, treatment, and prevention. Digitization affects all elements of the healthcare system. It changes the work of physicians and other medical professionals and alters the way health services are provided, thereby affecting patients through innovative medical treatment and possibly bringing additional prevention outcomes. Digital innovations in the health sector motivate hospitals and clinics to introduce new work processes and ultimately, create new approaches to health policy.

The main objective of this chapter is to map the research field dealing with digital innovations in health-related activities and identify current trends in this domain, including the most important thematic areas as well as the main countries contributing to research in this field, and provide the definition of digital health innovations along with their taxonomy. We conducted a bibliometric analysis of publications in this area in order to identify streams of research, and the most influential papers that discuss digital innovative solutions in health. It is followed by the systematic literature review focused on digital innovations in health. The chapter seeks to answer the following research questions (RQ):

RQ1: What are the trends in research on digital health innovations, including the impact of this research?

RQ2: Which are the main international contributing countries and institutions in digital health innovations research?

RQ3: What are the key research themes, how do they cluster, and what are the contexts of this research?

RQ4: How are digital health innovations defined in various scientific disciplines, and how can they be taxonomized?

DOI: 10.4324/9781032726557-3

Methodology and Data

The data used in a bibliometric analysis is retrieved from the Web of Science database. We searched titles, abstracts, and keywords of articles and review articles published in English using the following keywords selected on the basis of the WHO reports on digital health (e.g., WHO, 2021): "digital innovation+health*" OR "innovation*+ehealth*" OR "innovation*+e-health*" OR "innovation*+telemedicine" OR "Internet of Things+health*" OR "innovation+digital health*" OR "blockchain+health*" OR "big data+health*" OR "artificial intelligence+health*" OR "digital technology+health*" OR "innovation+digital treatment+health" OR "innovation+mhealth*" OR "digital innovation+healthcare."

Such a search brought 193 papers published in English in the years from January 1, 2014 to January 1, 2023, and when limited to articles and review articles, the sample consisted of 179 papers. We analyzed the content of the papers' abstracts and eliminated papers that were not relevant to our topic, thus reducing our sample to 142 articles. The process of the sample selection is presented in Table 1.1.

We studied this selected dataset with the use of a bibliometric methodology, i.e., applying mathematical and statistical methods and tools to analyze written communication (Pritchard, 1969; Yalcin & Daim, 2021). We performed analyses of keywords (including co-occurrence), co-authorship, bibliographic coupling and citations using the R software and the Vosviewer software tools. The latter allowed us to identify the most influential papers covering 49 papers with high (15 papers, 10.6%) and medium (34 papers, 24%) numbers of

Table 1.1 Data selection process

Data Source	WoS Database
Searching period	January 1, 2014 to January 1, 2023
Subject categories	"digital innovation+health*" OR "innovation*+ehealth*" OR "innovation*+e-health*" OR "innovation*+telemedicine" OR "Internet of Things+health*" OR "innovation+digital health*" OR "blockchain+healh*" OR "big data+health*" OR "artificial intelligence+health*" OR "digital technology+health*" OR "innovation+digital treatment+health" OR "innovation+mhealth*" OR "digital innovation+healthcare"
Language	English
Initial sample size	193
Document types	Articles or review articles
Sample size	179
Final sample size selected on the basis of content analysis of the abstracts	142

Source: Authors' elaboration based on Web of Science (WoS) database.

citations. These papers were further studied using the systematic literature review method as outlined by Kraus et al. (2022).

Bibliometric methodology

The main measure of impact used in this study is each paper's number of citations, normalized by the age of the paper. We conduct this normalization by subtracting the publication year from 2024, so that the minimum value is 1. Once we have this score in hand, we proceed to conduct four separate analyses.

The first simply examines the properties of this measure. In particular, we are interested in which values can be considered to be "high," and to make appropriate ranges that represent high and low values. We ultimately sort the papers into three groups of uneven size, which represent high, medium, and low numbers of citations per year.

Next, we examine which journals published the papers in each group. We note whether a single journal published multiple papers within each group – perhaps there is a source of high-impact papers, or one with a demonstrably worse record of success.

Third, we perform a keyword analysis, looking for common occurrences in each group. This is done by extracting and sorting the user-defined terms, with a necessary visual step where similar terms ("Internet of Things" vs. "Internet of Things (IoT)," for example) might be missed by purely mechanical methods. After noting the most common keywords in each group, co-occurrences are analyzed using the VOSviewer software tool.

Finally, we examine the countries of each author. We extract these from the affiliations in each paper and look for unique occurrences (i.e., two authors from the same country count as one). These are then aggregated by group, pooling the unique country occurrences from all papers into a single list. The most common countries, measured by share of the total in the list, are further analyzed.

Results of the Bibliometric Analysis

The bibliometric analysis allows to map various research fields that deal with digital health innovations. The first research step to address the RQ1 (*What are the trends in research on digital health innovations including the impact of this research?*) looking at the changes in the number of papers published since 2014. In the years 2013–2023, 193 scientific publications on digital innovations were published in all disciplines, out of which 179 were articles or review articles, with a number of publications growing sharply, especially since 2018 (Figure 1.1).

As is shown in Figure 1.2, the number of citations is heavily skewed toward the left. The median value is 1.5 cites per year. Of the 142 papers,

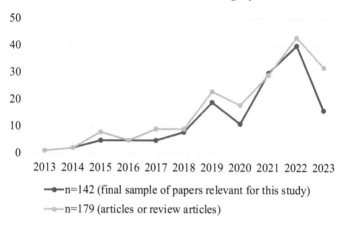

n=142 (final sample of papers relevant for this study)
n=179 (articles or review articles)

Figure 1.1 Number of papers on digital health innovations in the Web of Science database by year of publication in 2014–2023.

Source: Authors' work based on WoS data selected according to the criteria described in Table 1.1.

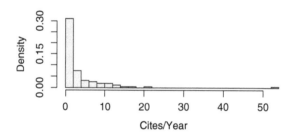

Figure 1.2 Distribution of citations per year

Source: Authors' work based on WoS data.

27 have no citations at all, and 62 have one or fewer. There is only one outlier far above the next highest value.

Visually examining the breakpoints in the sorted data, we find useful (and rather round) thresholds of 9.5 and 2.5. This gives us groups of 15 "high"-impact papers (10.6% of the total), along with 34 (24%) that can be classified as "medium" and 93 (65.5%) as "low."

The mean values for paper age (in years) in the high, medium, and low groupings are 4.53, 4.35, and 3.4 cites per year, respectively. Here, we see that there is no appreciable difference, particularly between the top two groups. Highly cited papers are not likely to be very old (representing accumulated impact) or very new (in which "fresh" papers get more attention).

Papers that are dedicated to summarizing and synthesizing the previous literature are particularly prized when writing one's own original research.

As such, they are often cited in subsequent work. Within each group, many of the highest-cited papers are classified as reviews, with 26.7, 8.8, and 14.0% of papers labeled as such in the high-, medium-, and low-citation categories. Here, the prevalence of review papers among the most-cited papers is of particular note.

Are any particular journals likely to be the most cited? Or the least cited? While most journals appear only once in each group, Table 1.2 shows which ones are represented two or more times. There does not appear to be any particular pattern. Nor does any particular journal make up a large percentage of the total. (The highest number, 4, is among 93 low-impact journals.)

Next, we examine common keywords. Since each paper has more than one, the size of the sample is larger. In Table 1.3, even the common keywords (matching *n* specific mentions plus *m* similar matches) make up small proportions of the total.

Which countries provide the most authors in each group of publications? Table 1.4 presents the highest proportions among the aggregated affiliations. China has the largest share in all three groups; this proportion is roughly ten times the average value for the medium and low-ranked groups. In the high-rank group, it is slightly less, leaving room for larger contributions by those countries that are ranked third through fifth. The US is regularly in second place, behind China, in all groups. India is regularly in third or fourth place. Of the rest, England appears in the highest and lowest categories.

Table 1.2 Journals with multiple appearances in each group

Journal's Rank	
High-Rank	
IEEE TRANSACTIONS ON INDUSTRIAL INFORMATICS	2
Medium-Rank	
IEEE JOURNAL OF BIOMEDICAL AND HEALTH INFORMATICS	2
JMIR MEDICAL INFORMATICS	2
SUSTAINABILITY	2
Low-Rank	
INTERNATIONAL JOURNAL OF ENVIRONMENTAL RESEARCH AND PUBLIC HEALTH	4
SENSORS	3
ACS APPLIED MATERIALS & INTERFACES	2
COMPUTERS IN BIOLOGY AND MEDICINE	2
DIGITAL HEALTH	2
FRONTIERS IN PUBLIC HEALTH	2
IEEE ACCESS	2
INTERNATIONAL JOURNAL OF COMPUTER SCIENCE AND NETWORK SECURITY	2
JMIR MHEALTH AND UHEALTH	2
JOURNAL OF RESPONSIBLE INNOVATION	2
LANCET DIGITAL HEALTH	2
RESULTS IN PHYSICS	2

Source: Authors' work based on WoS data.

Table 1.3 Common keywords by group

Group	Size	Common Keywords
High	71	Privacy (3+1)
Medium	175	data mining (4)
		healthcare (5+4)
Low	489	artificial intelligence (7+1)
		big data (10+3)
		digital health (5)
		Digitalization (5)
		healthcare (10+6)
		health information (9)
		Internet of Things (9)
		mHealth (6)
		Privacy (4+3)

Source: Authors' work based on WoS data.

Table 1.4 Countries with the highest proportions of author affiliations

High-rank	Prop.	Medium-rank	Prop.	Low-rank	Prop.
Peoples R China	0.333	Peoples R China	0.353	Peoples R China	0.237
US	0.200	US	0.294	US	0.215
India	0.200	India	0.118	England	0.129
Canada	0.133	Italy	0.118	India	0.086
England	0.133	Saudi Arabia	0.088	Netherlands	0.086
Means	0.0476		0.0345		0.0238

Source: Authors' work based on WoS data.

One potentially fruitful avenue for future research would be a gravity-type model, where factors such as economic or population size, a history with the English language, and other factors might describe these proportions.

Thematic and Network Analysis

To address the third research question (*RQ3: What are the key research themes, how do they cluster, and what are the contexts of this research?*), the final sample of 142 papers was selected as relevant to the topic based on the content analysis. It was then grouped according to the co-occurrence of keywords taking into consideration the strength of links. Thus, two thematic clusters of keywords were identified with 23 common keywords of total links strength equaled to 28. They are dominated by threads related to the type of digital technology (Figure 1.3):

• Thematic cluster 1 (grey) focused on Health Internet of Things (HIoT)
• Thematic cluster 2 (black), which is centered around big data and artificial intelligence (AI) usage in healthcare (in particular, machine learning and health informatics)

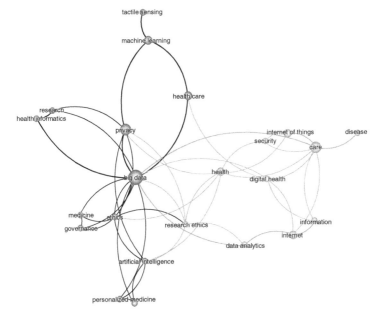

Figure 1.3 The most important research themes centered around digital health innovations: the analysis of the co-occurrence of keywords in publications indexed in the WoS database in 2014–2023 (n=142)

Note: Minimum cluster size=10 items

Source: Authors' elaboration of WoS data using VOSviewer software.

The identification of these two thematic clusters indicates the direction of our further study on digital innovations carried out in the literature review section.

Main Findings from the Literature Review

This section presents the main findings from the systematic literature review of 49 papers (i.e., 35%) in our sample that were highly cited. The aim is to answer the RQ4 (*How are digital health innovations defined in various scientific disciplines, and how can they be taxonomized?*).

It seems to be commonly understood what digital innovation is as only six papers in our sample try to define this phenomenon, either providing own definition or citing the definition of others. These definitions can be divided into wide ones, which try to cover the whole spectrum of digital technologies, or narrow ones focused only on specific technologies (telemedicine, Health IoT, etc.) (Table 1.5).

It seems to be too early to create a unique taxonomy of digital health innovations as the literature on this topic is still fragmented, and examples studied

Table 1.5 Definitions of digital innovation in health

Author(s)	Definition
Narrow approach to the definition	
Giacalone et al. (2018, p. 2)	"Big Data healthcare is conceived as a real digital collection of all that the patient has had, taken or required in the medical field"
Hossain and Muhammad (2016, p. 192)	"Health IoT is a combination of communication technologies, interconnected apps, Things (devices and sensors), and people that would function together as one smart system to monitor, track, and store patients' healthcare information for ongoing care."
Boccalandro et al. (2019, p. 385)	Telemedicine defined as "the distant supply of healthcare services and clinical assistance using information and communication technologies, such as the internet, wireless systems, and mobile phones" (definition of the American Telemedicine Association).
Wide approach to the definition	
Daher et al. (2017, p. 2)	Digital innovation such as electronic health (eHealth) encompasses non-internet and internet-enabled mHealth as well as other internet-based health interventions.
Egan (2020, pp. 2–3)	The use of digital technologies in disease monitoring, data analytics, diagnosis, treatments, accessing healthcare information, education, and support.
Iyanna et al. (2022, p. 151)	Digitally driven technological transformations occurring in diagnostics and equipment, in healthcare administration, management, and delivery.
Tromp et al. (2022)	Digital health solutions seek to address the health system challenges and can reflect client or provider-facing technologies and data services.

by scholars so far are still diverse, so the most appropriate is to apply the standard classification of innovations. Taking a closer look at the above definitions and some examples given in the literature, one can identify two digital innovation types as outlined by the OECD/Eurostat (2018): radical health innovations and incremental ones. It should be noted that digital innovations in health are mainly radical. This type of innovation predominates in both health products and health services.

Radical innovations transform the existing state of play, sometimes the disruptive solutions could be applied in a niche market at the beginning, and with time they diffuse throughout the market, eventually displacing solutions existing on the market (Christensen, 1997; OECD/Eurostat, 2018). The examples of this innovation type in the health sector that can be found in the literature include goods or services such as artificial intelligent optoelectronic skin integrating electronic and photonic functions (Gong et al., 2022), genomic analysis using AI (Abdelhalim et al., 2022), pressure-sensitive electronic skin and pressure sensors (Asghar et al., 2020), big data based diagnosis and treatments (Giacalone et al., 2018), biomedical data collection and analysis through smartphone app (Bahmani et al., 2021), and many others.

Incremental innovations, in turn, mean gradual improvements implemented on existing products or services (OECD/Eurostat, 2018). In the health sector, they are, for example, big databases integrating different types of medical data (Abdelhalim et al., 2022), electronic health records telemonitoring or remote monitoring for patients with cardiovascular diseases (Tromp et al., 2022), Internet used for health data transmission (Rubbio et al., 2018), or iPad-compatible language translation apps in healthcare (Panayiotou et al., 2019).

It is worth noting that majority of digital health innovations studied in the literature appear in healthcare services, e.g., remote patient monitoring systems with blockchain and IoT (Qahtan et al., 2022), big data analytics service that allows specifying the probability of a specific disease on each patient (Chawla & Davis, 2013), telemedicine services for patients with hemophilia (Boccalandro et al., 2019), Genomic analysis using AI (Abdelhalim et al., 2022).

Conclusions

The main conclusions from the review of relevant literature focused on digital health innovations can be summarized as follows:

- There are various definitions and approaches to digital innovation in health ranging from narrow ones by technology used, by type of health-related activities digitalized (products, processes, business models) to wider ones trying to cover all digital technologies and types of activities in healthcare and the health sector as a whole. However, a commonly accepted definition has not been elaborated so far.
- There are two main health-related areas where digital innovations are introduced: medical goods (product innovations) and medical services (mainly service product innovation, rarely business process innovations).
- Digital innovations in health are mainly radical; this type of innovation predominates in both health products and health services.

The bibliometric analysis conducted here shows that, although review papers do tend to be cited more frequently, there is no single journal that produces a high proportion of citations. Likewise, there are no "magic" keywords that are mentioned more frequently. The only significant pattern we uncovered is by country of authorship, with China, the US, and often India producing the most publications in this area.

This leads to a potentially fruitful line of future research: an empirical estimation of the determinants of productivity, as measured by citations. Since the largest countries seem to be most responsible, perhaps a gravity-type model would control for size in this fashion. At the same time, such a model could be extended to examine bilateral partnerships to explain which pairs are most likely to collaborate on e-health research.

References

Abdelhalim, H., Berber, A., Lodi, M., Jain, R., Nair, A., Pappu, A., Patel, K., Venkat, V., Venkatesan, C., Wable, R., Dinatale, M., Fu, A., Iyer, V., Kalove, I., Kleyman, M., Koutsoutis, J., Menna, D., Paliwal, M., Patel, N., Patel, T., Rafique, Z., Samadi, R., Varadhan, R., Bolla, S., Vadapalli, S., & Ahmed, Z. (2022). Artificial intelligence, healthcare, clinical genomics, and pharmacogenomics approaches in precision medicine. *Frontiers in Genetics, 13*, 929736. https://doi.org/10.3389/fgene.2022.929736

Asghar, W., Li, F., Zhou, Y., Wu, Y., Yu, Z., Li, S., Tang, D., Han, X., Shang, J., Liu, Y. W., & Li, R.-W. (2020). Piezocapacitive flexible e-skin pressure sensors having magnetically grown microstructures. *Advanced Materials Technologies, 5*, 1900934. https://doi.org/10.1002/admt.201900934

Bahmani, A., Alavi, A., Buergel, T., Upadhyayula, S., Wang, Q., Ananthakrishnan, S. K., Alavi, A., Celis, D., Gillespie, D., Young, G., Xing, Z., Nguyen, M. H. H., Haque, A., Mathur, A., Payne, J., Mazaheri, G., Li, K. J., Kotipalli, P., Liao, L., Bhasin, R., Cha, K., Rolnik, B., Celli, A., Dagan-Rosenfeld, O., Higgs, E., Zhou, W., Berry, C. L., Van Winkle, K. G., Contrepois, K., Ray, U., Bettinger, K., Datta, S., Li, X., & Snyder, M. P. (2021). A scalable, secure, and interoperable platform for deep data-driven health management. *Nature Communications, 12*, 5757. https://doi.org/10.1038/s41467-021-26040-1

Boccalandro, E. A., Dallari, G., & Mannucci, P. M. (2019). Telemedicine and telerehabilitation: Current and forthcoming applications in haemophilia. *Blood Transfusion, 17*, 385–390. https://doi.org/10.2450/2019.0218-18.

Chawla, N. V., & Davis, D. A. (2013). Bringing big data to personalized healthcare: A patient-centered framework. *Journal of General Internal Medicine, Suppl 3*, S660–S665. https://doi.org/10.1007/s11606-013-2455-8

Christensen, C. (1997). *The Innovator's Dilemma*. Harvard Business School Press, Cambridge, MA.

Daher, J., Vijh, R., Linthwaite, B., Dave, S., Kim, J., Dheda, K., Peter, T., & Pai, N. P. (2017). Do digital innovations for HIV and sexually transmitted infections work? Results from a systematic review (1996–2017). *BMJ Open, 7*, e017604. https://doi.org/10.1136/bmjopen-2017-017604

Egan, K. (2020). Digital technology, health and well-being and the Covid-19 pandemic: It's time to call forward informal carers from the back of the queue. *Seminars in Oncology Nursing, 36*, 151088.

Giacalone, M., Cusatellib, C., & Santarcangelo, V. (2018). Big data compliance for innovative clinical models. *Big Data Research, 12*, 35–40. https://doi.org/10.1016/j.bdr.2018.02.001

Gong, Y., Zhang, Y-Z., Fang, S., Liu, Ch., Niu, J., Li, G., Li, F., Li, Y., Cheng, T., & Lai W-Y. (2022) Artificial intelligent optoelectronic skin with anisotropic electrical and optical responses for multi-dimensional sensing. *Applied Physics Reviews, 9*(2), 021403. https://doi.org/10.1063/5.0083278

Hossain, M. S., & Muhammad, G. (2016). Cloud-assisted industrial Internet of Things (IIoT) – Enabled framework for health monitoring. *Computer Networks, 101*, 192–202. https://doi.org/10.1016/j.comnet.2016.01.009

Iyanna, S., Kaur, P., Ractham, P., Talwar, S., & Najmul Islam, A. K. M. (2022). Digital transformation of healthcare sector. What is impeding adoption and continued usage of technology-driven innovations by end-users? *Journal of Business Research, 153*, 150–161. https://doi.org/10.1016/j.jbusres.2022.08.007

Kraus, S., Breier, M., Lim, W. M., Dabić, M., Kumar, S., Kanbach, D., Mukherjee, D., Corvello, V., Piñeiro-Chousa, J., Liguori, E., Palacios-Marqués, D., Schiavone, F., Ferraris, A., Fernandes, C., & Ferreira, J. J. (2022). Literature reviews as independent studies: Guidelines for academic practice. *Review of Managerial Science, 16*, 2577–2595. https://doi.org/10.1007/s11846-022-00588-8

OECD/Eurostat (2018). *Oslo Manual 2018: Guidelines for collecting, reporting and using data on innovation, 4th edition. The measurement of scientific, technological and innovation activities.* OECD Publishing, Paris/Eurostat, Luxembourg, https://doi.org/10.1787/9789264304604-en

Panayiotou, A., Gardner, A., Williams, S., Zucchi, E., Mascitti-Meuter, M., Goh, A. M. Y., You, E., Chong, T. W. H., Logiudice, D., Lin, X., Haralambous, B., & Batchelor, F. (2019). Language translation apps in health care settings: Expert opinion. *JMIR Mhealth Uhealth, 7*(4), e11316. https://mhealth.jmir.org/2019/4/e11316/. https://doi.org/10.2196/11316

Pritchard, A. (1969). Statistical bibliography or bibliometrics. *Journal of Documentation, 25*, 348–349.

Qahtan, S., Khaironi, Y. S., Zaidan, A. A., Alsattar, H. A., Albahri, O. S., Zaidan, B. B., Zulzalil, H., Osman, M. H., Alamoodi, A. H., & Mohammed, R. T. (2022). Novel multi security and privacy benchmarking framework for blockchain-based IoT healthcare industry 4.0 systems. *IEEE Transactions on Industrial Informatics, 18*(9), 6415–6423. https://doi.org/10.1109/TII.2022.3143619

Rubbio, I., Bruccoleri, M., Pietrosi, A., & Ragonese, B. (2018). Digital health technology enhances resilient behaviour: Evidence from the ward. *International Journal of Operations & Production Management, 40*(1), 34–67. https://doi.org/10.1108/IJOPM-02-2018-0057

Tromp, J., Jindal, D., Redfern, J., Bhatt, A., Séverin, T., Banerjee, A., Ge, J., Itchhapora, D., Jaarsma, T., Lanas, F., Lopez-Jimenez, F., Mohamed, A., Perel, P., Perez, G. E., Pinto, F., Vedanthan, R., Verstrael, A., Yeo, K. K., Zulfiya, K., Prabhakaran, D., Lam, C. S. P., & Cowie, M. R. (2022). World Heart Federation roadmap for digital health in cardiology. *Global Heart, 17*(1), 61. https://doi.org/10.5334/gh.1141

WHO. (2021). *Global Strategy on Digital Health 2020-2025.* Geneva: World Health Organization.

Yalcin, H., & Daim, T. (2021). A scientometric review of technology capability research. *Journal of Engineering and Technology Management, 62*, 01658.

2 Digital Readiness in Healthcare

Comparative Analysis of EU and US Resources and Capabilities

Arkadiusz Michał Kowalski,
Małgorzata Stefania Lewandowska
and Dawid Majcherek

Introduction

Equal access to health services is considered a right of every citizen, however, despite the constitutional guarantee and governments' efforts to equalize access to publicly financed medical services, this access is still uneven and limited (González & Triunfo, 2020). The issue of healthcare access barriers is multifaceted, as patients encounter various challenges in accessing health services. These challenges could be alleviated through the implementation of digital health solutions. Thus, the objective of this chapter is to assess the readiness to use digital technologies in accessing healthcare services in European countries as well as in the US. There is an urgent need to learn from the experience of the COVID-19 pandemic, where digital health innovations were rapidly integrated and scaled to address challenges in healthcare delivery. However, there are many barriers related to the digitization of healthcare systems, both on the part of healthcare providers and their customers (patients). The rapid implementation of innovative solutions may lead to health disparities, characterized by variations in health outcomes and disproportionate allocation of healthcare resources across different demographic groups (Yao et al., 2022). In pursuit of the stated objective, we present an analysis of medical service access in EU countries and assess their level of digitization. In this context, an important part of the study is recommendations on how to make digital health solutions an effective way of providing health services to people in need, as well as coordinating the management of the healthcare system. Our research is based mostly on macroeconomic data, mainly public and private expenditure on healthcare in GDP, human and infrastructure resources with a focus on data on the number of physicians and hospital beds per capita, as well as data on quality of healthcare delivery and healthy lifestyle of society, and the level of digitalization. This chapter is structured as follows. The first

DOI: 10.4324/9781032726557-4

section reviews the literature on digitalization of the healthcare system. Next, country-level data sources used in this research are presented. This is followed by a presentation of the results of the analysis. The last section contains conclusions, together with recommendations for actions needed to increase healthcare digitalization in the analyzed regions.

Literature Review

In today's world, Europe faces four significant challenges in terms of healthcare: (i) the rise in chronic diseases, coupled with an aging population and rising societal demands; (ii) the influence of external environmental factors such as climate change; (iii) inequalities in access to healthcare; and (iv) the risk of losing the ability to protect populations from infectious disease threats, such as the COVID pandemic (European Commission, 2020). As a result, European policy aims to encourage the development of innovative interventions that are safer and more effective while also maintaining the goal of keeping older people active and independent for a longer time. Additionally, this helps to ensure the long-term viability of health and care delivery systems (Lewandowska, 2022). The decline in the number of persons employed, population, and labor productivity, all of which contribute to an increase in public spending, are some of the barriers that stand in the way of attaining these goals (European Commission, 2017).

Access to healthcare is a complex issue, and there are many different ways to conceptualize it. A peculiarity of the health services market is that the location of medical entities representing the supply does not correspond to the locally occurring demand. Healthcare availability may be viewed as a function of both demand and supply factors, such as the burden of disease and knowledge, attitudes, and self-care behaviors. Supply factors include the location, availability, cost, and appropriateness of services. Based on research conducted in the UK, the so-called *inverse care law* was formulated, according to which the availability of healthcare services in a region is inversely proportional to the size of the needs of the population living there (Tudor Hart, 2000). For example, the problem of uneven distribution of treatment capacity across Poland was identified in a NIK report (Naczelna Izba Kontroli, 2018), but a similar situation also exists in many other countries. Digital technologies serve as an aid in combatting inequality in access to medical services. Telemedicine solutions have the advantage of not requiring the presence of both parties, i.e., the medical entity and the patient, at the same time and in the same place. As a result, digital technologies increase the availability of medical services, especially in regions struggling with a deficit of inpatient healthcare (Czerwinska, 2015).

Even though digital health is a crucial strategic objective at the European Union level, aligned with the European Strategic Plan 2019–2024 as outlined by the European Commission, a problem affecting disparities in access to healthcare services is digital health inequalities, understood as differences in access, use, and effectiveness of digital technologies for health monitoring, diagnosis and treatment of diseases between different social groups (Libura, 2023). The healthcare industry still exhibits a much lower level of digital innovation in comparison to other sectors, such as the financial sector, the insurance sector, the retail sector, and media, which is a factor that limits growth in healthcare industry labor productivity (Gopal et al., 2019; Stoumpos et al., 2023).

There are five elements of access to healthcare services, as defined by Penchansky and Thomas: it has to be adequate (care should be continually tailored to the needs of patients), accessible (treatment is available at all stages of patient care, beginning with preventive/health services and progressing through all therapies, including non-medical assistance), affordable (individuals can get healthcare without getting into financial difficulty), appropriate (as healthcare must be inclusive, services must be applicable to the health requirements of various communities or groups), and available (all patients should have access to healthcare, including specialized treatments and any other service that contributes to high-quality healthcare) (Penchansky & Thomas, 1981).

Patients require access to healthcare services in the broadest sense possible, which includes access to a variety of different services relevant to their personal health, including digital innovation (European Patient Forum, 2016). When examining the concept of core preparedness for e-health solutions, many scholars primarily emphasize the recognition of needs or issues, and articulate discontentment with the current state of affairs (Kruszyńska-Fischbach et al., 2022). Digital readiness in healthcare concerns the preparedness of healthcare systems, institutions, and professionals to adopt and effectively use digital technologies to improve healthcare delivery. Hence, digital readiness can enhance access to healthcare by providing more opportunities for delivering care.

The term *effectiveness*, as employed by Campbell et al., pertains to the inclination of participants to ascertain whether e-health solutions would effectively fulfill a functional requirement in their professional practice prior to committing their resources, both in terms of time and finances, to implement a change (2001). However, the most important prerequisite for the functioning of the market for remote medical services is the development of the information society and the inclusion of all its members (Fundacja SeniorApp, 2023). When some digital health innovations, however, could not be sustained over time, many digital health interventions were stopped. In contrast to how quickly digital transformations are developing, it may take years for a change to be approved by the authorities (van Velthoven et al., 2019). Hospitals should therefore accurately identify their Industry 4.0 and digital transformation preparations and, after determining their needs, set up road maps defining the actions they must take to raise their current level. Bilgiç et al. determined the criteria that affect the concept of digital transformation in healthcare created and validated a model based on these criteria, grouped under five main factors: management support, current status tracking, corporate culture, resource reservation, and service management (Bilgiç & Camgöz Akdağ, 2023).

One of the most important factors determining the availability of healthcare services is medical personnel, who influence the effective functioning of the entire healthcare system. Doctors and other medical professionals are responsible for healthcare, which is one of the greatest assets of man and society as a whole. The development and maintenance of a country's medical personnel, as well as the overall functioning of the healthcare system, is heavily dependent on public spending on healthcare. This spending makes it possible not only to meet current health needs but also to address long-term *grand challenges* related to critical health and development issues, including population aging and diseases of civilization (Kowalski, 2022).

Digital technologies provide an opportunity to further increase the efficiency of healthcare systems. Healthcare is undergoing a digital transformation that eliminates the inefficient steps in the process and creates a more productive environment (Bilgiç & Camgöz Akdağ, 2023). Telemedicine solutions enable rapid communication between patients and healthcare providers and the transfer of data (such as test results) between different players in the healthcare market, as well as direct contact between patients and healthcare professionals. These include e-counselling, electronic records, health information networks, health information on the Internet and electronic registries, portable devices used to monitor the body's condition, and an electronic unified system for monitoring queues, allowing patients to find an appointment with a specialist or an examination date faster than by traditional means. Digitalization helps to increase the quality, accessibility, and efficiency of healthcare services on the one hand, and to lower healthcare costs on the other. From a macroeconomic point of view, telemedicine leads to economic growth by affecting productivity levels and competitiveness in healthcare (Czerwinska, 2015).

Indeed, digital technologies can play a key role in transforming the healthcare system and making it more functional and efficient. The use of these technologies will make it possible to increase the quality of healthcare services to the benefit of both patients and medical personnel. This is because telemedicine solutions make it possible to monitor a patient's condition regardless of their physical location – in or out of the hospital. In turn, data on the patient's condition can be transferred between the patient and the doctor and centers that care for patients. In this way, digital solutions help to eliminate the gap in access to healthcare. The main goals of digitization in the healthcare system include optimizing the work of doctors, improving patient outcomes, reducing human error, and lowering costs (Schrijvers, 2017). Digitalization can also optimize cooperation between the hub hospitals and hospitals located in the more remote areas (Modern Helathcare Institute, 2023).

Universal access to medical care, considered a right of every citizen, should therefore depend primarily on need, not on the ability to pay for it.

Despite the constitutional guarantee and measures taken by governments to level the playing field in access to publicly funded medical services, especially in the case of underdeveloped countries, access is still unequal and limited (González & Triunfo, 2020).

While the waiting time for a medical appointment is closely related to the capacity of the healthcare system, the inability to cover the cost of treatment remains primarily a result of a patient's low-income level. Raittio et al., studying the level of dental care in Finland, refer to this problem as *income-related inequality* (Raittio et al., 2016) while González and Triunfo, analyzing the performance of the healthcare system in Uruguay, describe this condition explicitly as *pro-rich inequality* (González & Triunfo, 2020).

Data and Methods

Identification of resources and capabilities as well as barriers in implementation of various digital innovations in the healthcare sector requires a multidimensional perspective.

This research includes macroeconomic data (public and private spending on healthcare in GDP), human and infrastructure resources (including the number of physicians and hospital beds per capita), quality of healthcare delivery and healthy lifestyle of society (measured by healthy life expectancy in years), and digitalization (using the Internet to seek health information on the Internet and introducing electronic medical records).

The following country-level data sources were used for this analysis:

– Domestic general government health expenditure (% of GDP) (World Bank, 2020a)
– Domestic private health expenditure (PVT-D) as a percentage of current health expenditure (CHE) (%) (World Health Organization, 2020b)
– Physicians (per 1,000 people) (World Health Organization, 2020a)
– Hospital beds (per 10 000 population) (World Health Organization, 2020c)
– Healthy life expectancy (HALE) at birth (years) (World Health Organization, 2019)
– Individuals using the Internet (% of population) (World Bank, 2020b)
– Percentage of inhabitants using the Internet to seek health information (Eurostat, 2022; Finney Rutten et al., 2019)
– Proportion of primary care medical practices using electronic medical records (OECD, 2021)

A comparative analysis between Central and Eastern Europe (CEE), the former European Union (EU-15), the European Union (all 27 countries), and the US was conducted. Descriptive statistics were calculated for the primary characteristics of the different regions. Furthermore, two-dimensional graphs that illustrated significant connections within the same data category were provided.

Results

Healthcare digitalization may lead to better access to medical services and higher patient satisfaction, especially for patients who face the most barriers to traditional face-to-face contact (due to age or traveling long distances).

However, there are numerous differences in healthcare access and digitalization readiness for the US and even within EU countries. This research presents the results for all EU countries in comparison to the US. Moreover, within EU countries, a sub-analysis was conducted for Central and Eastern Europe (12 countries defined in the Supplementary Materials Table S1), and EU-15 (the 15 pre-2004 EU Member States).

The level of per capita healthcare expenditure, which covers both public and private healthcare, depends on a mix of demographic, social, and economic factors. In 2020, the domestic general government healthcare expenditure in the US was 10.7% of GDP in comparison to 8.0% in EU countries. However, expenditure in Western European countries like Germany or France (see Supplementary files Table S1) is closer to US expenditure, while the average spending in the CEE regions is almost half that in the US (5.4% of GDP). Table 2.1 presents private healthcare expenditure as a percentage of current healthcare expenditure which do not differ between CEE and the EU-15 countries. However, the private healthcare expenditure in the US is almost double that in the EU (43.2% in US vs 24.5% in EU). Medicaid and Medicare continue to play an important role in purchasing healthcare in the US (OECD, 2021) while in Europe private insurance companies play a limited role.

Table 2.1 Summary statistics of data related to digital readiness and macroeconomic determinants

	US	*EU*	*EU-15*	*CEE*
Domestic general government health expenditure (% of GDP)	10.7%	8.0%	8.6%	5.4%
Domestic private health expenditure (PVT-D) as percentage of current health expenditure (CHE) (%)	43.2%	24.5%	24.3%	25.0%
Physicians (per 1,000 people)	2.6	3.9	4.2	3.1
Hospital beds (per 10,000 population)	28.7	53.9	50.4	65.5
Healthy life expectancy (HALE) at birth (years)	66.1	70.9	71.5	68.0
Individuals using the Internet (% of population)	91.8%	87.0%	87.4%	84.7%
% of inhabitants using Internet to seek health information	74.4%	52.2%	52.9%	49.4%
Proportion of primary care medical practices using electronic medical records	92.8%	79.1%	91.3%	37.4%

Source: Authors' work.

Both healthcare professionals (including physicians) and facilities (including hospital beds with proper geographic distribution) are crucial for addressing the health needs of society. The number of physicians per 1,000 inhabitants in the US is similar to CEE (2.6 vs 3.1 per 1,000 people). However, the EU-15 is more human resource-rich (4.2 physicians per 1,000 people). The further development of digital solutions requires healthcare workers to have the proper skills. Due to shortages of physicians in CEE and the US, this may cause a problem with training, time allocation, and effective implementation of digital platforms. The debate is ongoing about healthcare delivery through inpatient or outpatient care. In CEE, the healthcare model is more traditional, and many procedures are undertaken by way of hospitalization. This model is characterized by the highest number of hospital beds in CEE (65 beds per 10,000 inhabitants). In the EU-15, the number is 50 beds per 10,000 inhabitants, while in the US it is only 28 beds per 10,000 inhabitants. The EU-15 and US models focus on the reduction of the cost of a hospital stay. Digital follow-up after leaving hospital is a new opportunity for better capacity management of beds in hospital.

Healthy life expectancy (HALE) is one of the indicators measuring a country's health level. HALE is comprehensive indicators which reflect not only life expectancy but also quality of life. Surprisingly, the lowest HALE is 66.1 years in the US, which is lower by more than five years than in the EU-15 (71.5 years). Even for CEE countries, HALE is 68 years, which is higher than in the US.

In terms of digitalization of society, one in two EU citizens (53%) looked for health information online in 2022. This level is significantly lower than in the US, where almost 75% of citizens look for health information online. There difference between the CEE and EU-15 countries is only minor. Although there is no gap in overall Internet usage between the US and EU (91.8% vs 87.4%), the difference in the use of the Internet as a source of health information between US and EU citizens is more visible.

The last element related to digital readiness is the proportion of primary care medical practices using electronic medical records (EMR). In the US, almost 93% of primary care physicians use EMR, which is a similar level to the EU-15 countries (91.3%). However, there is a large gap in CEE countries, which seem to be less digitalized on the primary care level (only 37% of physicians use EMR).

Figure 2.1 presents healthy life expectancy in years on the vertical axis and domestic general government health expenditure as a percentage of GDP on the horizontal axis for all analyzed countries. CEE countries are presented as orange points, EU-15 countries as blue ones, and the US as a green point. The purple dotted lines present the EU average from Table 2.1. Figure 2.1 reveals that the majority of CEE countries' healthcare spending is significantly below the EU level, while healthy life expectancy in CEE is also below the EU level. The two exceptions are Greece and Cyprus, where HALE is above the

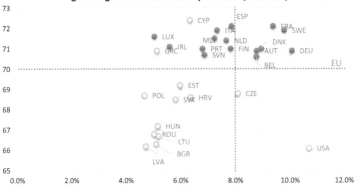

Figure 2.1 Countries in terms of healthy life expectancy (in years) and domestic general government health expenditure (% of GDP)

Source: Authors' work.

EU average regardless of public spending on healthcare being below the EU level. The lowest domestic government spending on healthcare is observed in Poland (4.72%), Latvia (4.67%), and Romania (5.02%). Low expenditure on healthcare is a huge barrier for creation and implementation of digital tools and training of healthcare professionals to use them effectively. The lowest HALE is measured in Latvia (66.2 years), Bulgaria (66.3 years), and Lithuania (66.7 years). For all EU-15 countries, HALE is above the EU average, while domestic general governmental health expenditure is above the EU average mainly for Western countries such as Germany, France, Denmark, Austria, Belgium, and Sweden (see Supplementary materials Table S1). The highest HALE among EU-15 countries is noted in Sweden (72.4 years), France (72.1 years), Spain (72.1 years), and Italy (71.9 years). There is a noticeable trend that lower government expenditure on healthcare in CEE countries results in lower life expectancy with good quality of life. Lower spending on healthcare reduces access to novel therapies and overall lower quality of patient care. However, although public and private healthcare expenditure is the highest in the US, healthy life expectancy does not reflect this. Thus, not only proper financing on healthcare is crucial to improve HALE. However, better financing for CEE countries should be a first step to ensure proper development of digital tools in order to improve digital readiness of healthcare professionals and patients.

Figure 2.2 presents healthy life expectancy in years on the vertical axis and the number of physicians per 1,000 people on the horizontal axis. Figure 2.2

shows that the number of doctors per capita was lowest in Poland, the US, Malta, Romania, and Luxembourg (see details in Supplementary materials Table S1). The numbers of physicians per capita for Greece, Austria, and Portugal are over-estimated, because they include all doctors licensed to practice (e.g., doctors in retirement). However, for a majority of CEE countries and the US, the lowest number of physicians may not only be an important barrier to implementing digital solutions. It also reduces HALE. An increase in the number of healthcare professionals in the US and CEE countries may be beneficial for waiting lists, quality of care, and in the long run for the digitalization of healthcare services.

Figure 2.3 presents the percentage of the population that uses the Internet to seek health information on the vertical axis and domestic private healthcare expenditure as a percentage of current healthcare expenditure on the horizontal axis. There are no significant differences within the EU between the EU-15 and CEE countries. Private healthcare expenditure does not correspond to the percentage of inhabitants using the Internet to seek health information. However, healthcare financing in the US requires private spending, thus citizens look for health information online more often than the EU population. The lowest private spending on healthcare is observed among citizens of Luxembourg (11.45% of current healthcare expenditure), the Czech Republic (12.58%), and Sweden (14.09%). The highest private healthcare expenditure is observed among CEE country citizens, particularly in Greece (45.88%), Bulgaria (38.13%), and Latvia (36.39%). As for digitalization of society, the highest percentage of citizens using the Internet to seek health information is in Denmark (98.87%), Luxembourg (98.66%), and Ireland (95.17%). Importantly, there is no significant difference in usage of the Internet to find health information among all of the EU countries, thus there should be no technological barrier to implementing digital solutions for both the EU and US population.

Figure 2.4 presents the percentage of the population using the Internet to seek health information on the vertical axis and overall Internet usage by the population on the horizontal axis. The lowest percentage of people using the Internet to seek health information is among citizens of Romania (28.9%), Germany (36.6%), and Bulgaria (39.1%). Finland (80.5%), the Netherlands (78%), and the US (74.4$) are the countries with the highest percentage of citizens who look for health information online. With a few exceptions, there is a visible trend in which overall Internet usage causes an increase in the use of the Internet to seek health information. Interestingly, most Western countries, such as Germany, France, Belgium, and Luxemburg, exceed the EU average (52%) in using the Internet as source of health information. Compared to the US, in Europe the barriers to searching for health information online need to be addressed.

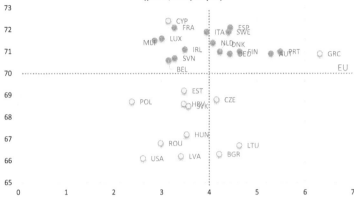

Figure 2.2 Countries in terms of healthy life expectancy (in years) and number of physicians (per 1,000 people)

Source: Author's work.

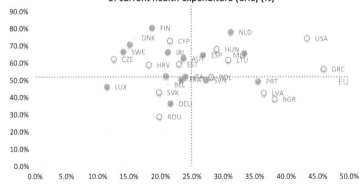

Figure 2.3 Countries according to percentage of the population using the Internet to
seek health information and domestic private healthcare expenditure as a
percentage of current healthcare expenditure

Source: Author's work.

Conclusions

One of the basic indicators showing the development of a healthcare system, which is per capita healthcare expenditure, covering both public and private healthcare expenditure, are the highest level in the US (10.7% of GDP, in comparison to 8.0% in EU countries). However, the European healthcare system is not homogeneous, with substantial variations in the level of its development across different countries. For example, Western European countries such as Germany and France exhibit a closer alignment with the US' expenditures, whereas the Central and Eastern European (CEE) regions demonstrate significantly lower average spending, amounting to nearly half of the US' expenditure as a percentage of their respective GDP (5.4%).

Regarding the digitalization of society, it was observed that approximately half of the European Union (EU) population, specifically 53% of EU citizens, engaged in the practice of accessing health-related information through online platforms in 2022. The prevalence of health information-seeking online is notably lower in this context, compared to the US, where approximately 75% of the population engages in such activities. There is a slight disparity between the Central and Eastern European (CEE) countries and the European Union-15 (EU-15) countries. While there is no discernible disparity in overall Internet usage rates between the US and the European Union, with rates of 91.8% and 87.4%, respectively, there is a more pronounced contrast in the use of the Internet as a source of health-related information among individuals residing in these regions.

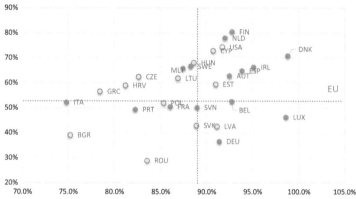

Figure 2.4 Countries in terms of percentage of the population using the Internet to seek health information and general Internet usage

Source: Author's work.

As for the primary care medical practices that use electronic medical records (EMR), in the US 93% of primary care physicians use electronic medical records (EMR), a proportion that is comparable to that of the EU-15 countries, which stands at 91.3%. Nevertheless, there is a significant disparity in the level of digitalization among Central and Eastern European (CEE) countries, particularly in the domain of primary care. Only 37% of physicians in these countries have adopted electronic medical records (EMR) systems. Based on the analysis, recommendations can be formulated for the actions needed to increase healthcare digitalization in the analyzed regions, presented in Table 2.2.

For all countries, as recommended by the World Health Organization, it is important to take into account the alignment of digital health performance monitoring criteria with a national and/or global action plan (World Health Organization, 2021, pp. 2020–2025).

Several recent studies showed that digitalization of healthcare reveals many barriers such as financial, legal, awareness-related, technological, and IT (Furlepa et al., 2022; LeRouge & Garfield, 2013). The first step toward development of digitalization of healthcare is elimination of those barriers. That is why our research shows that different regions in the EU require different approaches to elimination of obstacles. Although many studies focus on single or few countries' approach (Hyppönen et al., 2015; LeRouge & Garfield, 2013; Luciano et al., 2020), this study covers 27 EU countries and the US.

Furthermore, it is imperative that strategies pertaining to digital health are firmly rooted in the fundamental principles of the Sustainable Development Goals (SDG) and universal health coverage (UHC), which refers to the provision of comprehensive and high-quality healthcare services to all individuals, ensuring that they are accessible, delivered in a timely fashion, and free of financial constraints (Universal Health Coverage, 2023). These concepts, notably equity, solidarity, and human rights, should serve as the guiding framework for the implementation of digital health initiatives (Governing Health Futures 2030 Commission, 2021).

Table 2.2 Final recommendations for further healthcare digitalization in different regions

Region	Recommendations for Actions to Expand Healthcare Digitalization
US	Human resources (number of physicians per capita) with proper digital skills training
	Increase number of hospital beds with optimal capacity planning and human resources allocation
EU-15	Awareness campaign to encourage citizens to look for health information (including lifestyle) online
CEE	Increase domestic government expenditure on healthcare (% of GDP) including software, service and access to novel therapies
	Human resources (number of physicians per capita) with proper digital skills training
	Implementation of electronic medical records for healthcare professionals (mainly primary care physicians)

References

Bilgiç, D., & Camgöz Akdağ, H. (2023). Digital transformation readiness factors in healthcare. *Hospital Topics, 101*(3), 199–207. https://doi.org/10.1080/00185868.20 21.2002745

Campbell, J. D., Harris, K. D., & Hodge, R. (2001). Introducing telemedicine technology to rural physicians and settings. *The Journal of Family Practice, 50*(5), 419–424.

Czerwinska, M. (2015). Narzędzia e-zdrowia jako instrumenty poprawiające dostęp do usług medycznych w regionie (E-health tools as instruments to improve access to medical services in the region). *Nierówności Społeczne a Wzrost Gospodarczy, 3,* 173–185. https://doi.org/10.15584/nsawg.2015.3.14

European Commission. (2017). *Work programme 2016–2017.* https://ec.europa.eu/research/participants/data/ref/h2020/wp/2016_2017/main/h2020-wp1617-health_en.pdf.

European Commission. (2020). *Horizon 2020.* https://ec.europa.eu/programmes/horizon 2020/en/h2020-section/societal-challenges

European Patient Forum. (2016). *Defining and measuring access to healthcare: The patients' perspective.* https://www.eu-patient.eu/globalassets/policy/access/epf_position_defining_and_measuring_access_010316.pdf

Eurostat. (2022). *Internet use: Seeking health information.* https://ec.europa.eu/eurostat/databrowser/view/isoc_ci_ac_i/default/table?lang=en

Finney Rutten, L. J., Blake, K. D., Greenberg-Worisek, A. J., Allen, S. V., Moser, R. P., & Hesse, B. W. (2019). Online health information seeking among US adults: Measuring progress toward a healthy people 2020 objective. *Public Health Reports, 134*(6), 617–625. https://doi.org/10.1177/0033354919874074

Fundacja SeniorApp. (2023). *Polub się z telefonem. Cyfrowy świat jest prostszy niż myślisz. Poradnik dla senoora* [Computer software]. https://seniorapp.pl/polub-sie-z-telefonem-cyfrowy-swiat-jest-prostszy-niz-myslisz-poradnik-dla-seniora

Furlepa, K., Tenderenda, A., Kozłowski, R., Marczak, M., Wierzba, W., & Śliwczyński, A. (2022). Recommendations for the development of telemedicine in Poland based on the analysis of barriers and selected telemedicine solutions. *International Journal of Environmental Research and Public Health, 19*(3), Article 3. https://doi.org/10.3390/ijerph19031221

González, C., & Triunfo, P. (2020). Horizontal inequity in the use and access to health care in Uruguay. *International Journal for Equity in Health, 19*(1), 127. https://doi.org/10.1186/s12939-020-01237-w

Gopal, G., Suter-Crazzolara, C., Toldo, L., & Eberhardt, W. (2019). Digital transformation in healthcare – Architectures of present and future information technologies. *Clinical Chemistry and Laboratory Medicine (CCLM), 57*(3), 328–335. https://doi.org/10.1515/cclm-2018-0658

Governing Health Futures 2030 Commission. (2021). *Policy brief: Digital health futures readiness.* https://governinghealthfutures2030.org/pdf/policy-briefs/Digital-HealthFuturesReadiness.pdf

Hyppönen, H., Kangas, M., Reponen, J., Nohr, C., Villumsen, S., Koch, S., Hardardottir, G. A., Gilstad, H., Jerlvall, L., Pehrsson, T., Faxvaag, A., Anderssem, H., Brattheim, B., Vilmarlund, V., & Kaipio, J. (2015). *Nordic eHealth Benchmarking—Status 2014.* https://research.aalto.fi/en/publications/nordic-ehealth-benchmarking-status-2014

Kowalski, A. M. (2022). Healthcare systems and pharmaceutical industry in emerging and developed economies: China and Poland versus the US and the EU. In Weresa, M., Ciecierski, Ch., Filus, L. (Eds.) *Economics and Mathematical Modeling in Health-Related Research* (pp. 165–179). Brill. https://doi.org/10.1163/9789004517295_010

Kruszyńska-Fischbach, A., Sysko-Romańczuk, S., Napiórkowski, T. M., Napiórkowska, A., & Kozakiewicz, D. (2022). Organizational e-health readiness: How to prepare the primary healthcare providers' services for digital transformation. *International Journal of Environmental Research and Public Health, 19*(7), Article 7. https://doi.org/10.3390/ijerph19073973

LeRouge, C., & Garfield, M. J. (2013). Crossing the telemedicine chasm: Have the U.S. barriers to widespread adoption of telemedicine been significantly reduced? *International Journal of Environmental Research and Public Health, 10*(12), Article 12. https://doi.org/10.3390/ijerph10126472

Lewandowska, M. S. (2022). Meeting grand challenges: Assessment of Horizon 2020 Health, Demographic Change and Wellbeing projects. In Weresa, M., Ciecierski, Ch., Filus, L. (Eds.) *Economics and Mathematical Modeling in Health-Related Research* (pp. 121–145). Brill. https://doi.org/10.1163/9789004517295_008

Libura, M. (2023). Cyfrowe nierówności w zdrowiu. In Libera, M., Imiela, T., Głód Śliwińska, D. (Eds.) *Cyfryzacja zdrowia w interesie społecznym* (pp. 115–126). Okręgowa Izba Lekarska w Warszawie. https://izba-lekarska.pl/wp-content/uploads/2023/05/OIL_Cyfryzacja_raport_07042023.pdf

Luciano, E., Mahmood, M. A., & Mansouri Rad, P. (2020). Telemedicine adoption issues in the United States and Brazil: Perception of healthcare professionals. *Health Informatics Journal, 26*(4), 2344–2361. https://doi.org/10.1177/1460458220902957

Modern Healthcare Institute. (2023, September 4). Nie jestem optymistą. *mzdrowie.pl.* https://www.mzdrowie.pl/kadry/nie-jestem-optymista/

Naczelna Izba Kontroli. (2018). *System ochrony zdrowia w Polsce–stan obecny i pożądane kierunki zmian.* https://www.nik.gov.pl/plik/id,20223,vp,22913.pdf

OECD. (2021). *Health at a glance 2021: OECD indicators.* OECD. https://doi.org/10.1787/ae3016b9-en

Penchansky, R., & Thomas, J. W. (1981). The concept of access: Definition and relationship to consumer satisfaction. *Medical Care, 19*(2), 127–140. https://doi.org/10.1097/00005650-198102000-00001

Raittio, E., Aromaa, A., Kiiskinen, U., Helminen, S., & Suominen, A. L. (2016). Income-related inequality in perceived oral health among adult Finns before and after a major dental subsidization reform. *Acta Odontologica Scandinavica, 74*(5), 348–354. https://doi.org/10.3109/00016357.2016.1142113

Schrijvers, G. (2017). *Opieka koordynowana. Lepiej i taniej. Narodowy Fundusz Zdrowia, Warszawa.* https://koordynowana.nfz.gov.pl/wp-content/uploads/2022/05/Opieka-koordynowana-Lepiej-i-taniej-Guus-Schrijvers.pdf

Stoumpos, A. I., Kitsios, F., & Talias, M. A. (2023). Digital transformation in healthcare: Technology acceptance and its applications. *International Journal of Environmental Research and Public Health, 20*(4), 3407. https://doi.org/10.3390/ijerph20043407

Tudor Hart, J. (2000). Commentary: Three decades of the inverse care law. *BMJ (Clinical Research Ed.), 320*(7226), 18–19.

Universal Health Coverage. (2023). *UHC2030.* UHC2030. https://www.uhc2030.org/

van Velthoven, M. H., Cordon, C., & Challagalla, G. (2019). Digitization of health-care organizations: The digital health landscape and information theory. *International Journal of Medical Informatics, 124*, 49–57. https://doi.org/10.1016/j.ijmedinf.2019.01.007

World Bank. (2020a). *World development indicators.* https://databank.worldbank.org/source/world-development-indicators

World Bank. (2020b). *World telecommunication/ICT indicators database—Individuals using the Internet.* World Bank Open Data. https://data.worldbank.org

World Health Organization. (2019). *The global health observatory data—Healthy life expectancy (HALE).* WHO; World Health Organization. https://apps.who.int/gho/data/view.main.HALEXv

World Health Organization. (2020a). *Global Health Workforce Statistics.* World Bank Open Data. https://data.worldbank.org/indicator/SH.MED.PHYS.ZS

World Health Organization. (2020b). *The Global Health Observatory Data—Domestic Private Health Expenditure (PVT-D) as Percentage of Current Health Expenditure (CHE) (%).* https://www.who.int/data/gho/data/indicators/indicator-details/GHO/domestic-private-health-expenditure-(pvt-d)-as-percentage-of-current-health-expenditure-(che)-(-)

World Health Organization. (2020c). *The Global Health Observatory Data—Hospital Beds.* https://www.who.int/data/gho/data/indicators/indicator-details/GHO/hospital-beds-(per-10-000-population)

World Health Organization. (2021). *Global Strategy on Digital Health 2020–2025.* https://www.who.int/publications-detail-redirect/9789240020924

Yao, R., Zhang, W., Evans, R., Cao, G., Rui, T., & Shen, L. (2022). Inequities in health care services caused by the adoption of digital health technologies: Scoping review. *Journal of Medical Internet Research, 24*(3), e34144. https://doi.org/10.2196/34144

Appendix

Table S1 Database

Country Name	Region	Country Code	Domestic General Government Health Expenditure (% of GDP)	Domestic Private Health Expenditure (PVT-D) as Percentage a of Current Health Expenditure (CHE) (%)	Physicians (per 1,000 people)	Hospital Beds (per 10 000 population)	Healthy Life Expectancy (HALE) at Birth (years)	Individuals Using the Internet (% of population)	% of Inhabitants Using Internet to Seek Health Information	Proportion of Primary Care Medical Practices Using Electronic Medical Records
Bulgaria	CEE	BGR	5.1%	38.1%	4.2	74.5	66.3	75.3%	39.1%	NA
Croatia	CEE	HRV	6.4%	18.1%	3.5	55.4	68.6	81.3%	59.0%	NA
Czech Republic	CEE	CZE	8.1%	12.6%	4.2	66.2	68.8	82.7%	62.4%	86.0%
Estonia	CEE	EST	6.0%	22.9%	3.5	45.7	69.2	91.0%	59.5%	100.0%
Hungary	CEE	HUN	5.2%	28.9%	3.5	70.1	67.2	88.6%	68.1%	100.0%
Lithuania	CEE	LTU	5.2%	30.8%	4.6	64.3	66.7	86.9%	61.9%	100.0%
Latvia	CEE	LVA	4.7%	36.4%	3.4	54.9	66.2	91.2%	42.6%	77.0%
Poland	CEE	POL	4.7%	28.0%	2.4	65.4	68.7	85.4%	52.0%	30.3%
Romania	CEE	ROU	5.0%	19.8%	3.0	68.9	66.8	83.6%	28.9%	NA
Slovenia	CEE	SVN	6.9%	27.2%	3.3	44.3	70.7	89.0%	50.2%	100.0%
Slovakia	CEE	SVK	5.8%	19.7%	3.6	57.0	68.5	88.9%	43.0%	NA
Cyprus	CEE	CYP	6.3%	21.5%	3.1	34.0	72.4	90.8%	72.9%	NA
Austria	EU-15	AUT	8.8%	23.6%	5.3	72.7	70.9	92.5%	62.8%	80.0%
Belgium	EU-15	BEL	8.8%	20.8%	3.1	55.8	70.6	92.8%	52.6%	80.0%
Denmark	EU-15	DNK	8.9%	15.1%	4.2	26.0	71.0	98.9%	70.8%	100.0%

(Continued)

Table S1 (Continued)

Country Name	Region	Country Code	Domestic General Government Health Expenditure (% of GDP)	Domestic Private Health Expenditure (PVT-D) as Percentage a of Current Health Expenditure (CHE) (%)	Physicians (per 1,000 people)	Hospital Beds (per 10 000 population)	Healthy Life Expectancy (HALE) at Birth (years)	Individuals Using the Internet (% of population)	% of Inhabitants Using Internet to Seek Health Information	Proportion of Primary Care Medical Practices Using Electronic Medical Records
Finland	EU-15	FIN	7.8%	18.7%	4.6	36.1	71.0	92.8%	80.5%	NA
France	EU-15	FRA	9.4%	23.3%	3.3	59.1	72.1	86.1%	50.5%	80.0%
Germany	EU-15	DEU	10.1%	21.6%	4.4	80.0	70.9	91.4%	36.6%	100.0%
Greece	EU-15	GRC	5.1%	45.9%	6.3	42.0	70.9	78.5%	56.6%	100.0%
Ireland	EU-15	IRL	5.6%	21.2%	3.5	29.7	71.1	95.2%	66.3%	95.0%
Italy	EU-15	ITA	7.3%	23.9%	3.9	31.4	71.9	74.9%	52.2%	90.7%
Luxembourg	EU-15	LUX	5.0%	11.5%	3.0	42.6	71.6	98.7%	46.4%	99.0%
Malta	EU-15	MLT	7.2%	33.3%	2.9	44.9	71.5	87.5%	65.8%	NA
Netherlands	EU-15	NLD	7.7%	31.2%	4.1	31.7	71.4	92.1%	78.0%	100.0%
Portugal	EU-15	PRT	6.8%	35.5%	5.5	34.5	71.0	82.3%	49.5%	100.0%
Spain	EU-15	ESP	7.8%	26.7%	4.4	29.7	72.1	93.9%	64.9%	99.0%
Sweden	EU-15	SWE	9.8%	14.1%	4.4	21.4	71.9	88.3%	66.7%	100.0%
US	Non-EU	US	10.7%	43.2%	2.6	28.7	66.1	91.8%	74.4%	92.8%
Central & Eastern Europe	CEE	CEE	5.4%	25.0%	3.1	65.5	68.0	84.7%	49.4%	37.4%
15 pre-2004 EU Member States	EU-15	EU-15	8.6%	24.3%	4.2	50.4	71.5	87.4%	52.9%	91.3%
European Union (27 countries)	EU	EU	8.0%	24.5%	3.9	53.9	70.9	87.0%	52.2%	79.1%

Source: authors' work based on Eurostat, World Bank and World Health Organization data.

3 Funding of the Digital Health Transformation in the US

Comparative Study of Venture Capital and Initial Public Offering

Izabela Pruchnicka-Grabias

Introduction

A digital health revolution cannot happen without financial support. It is broadly financed by venture capital, and at a later stage this can be an initial public offering (IPO). Venture capital is a form of private financing, whereas in an IPO stocks are offered in a company to the public on stock exchanges.

The author analyses venture capital and initial public offerings, which are the most important means of financing. The development of digital health funding is studied, and this raises questions whether there is still financial potential to develop it. The data shows that 2021 was a record year as far as initial public offerings and venture capital fundings are concerned. The author examines whether these ways of gathering funds have prospects for further development. It is assumed that if there are investors interested in digital health stocks, it is possible to develop financing through stock exchanges. Furthermore, investors are interested if digital health stocks can be either diversifiers or hedgers or can replace other assets in a portfolio thanks to better risk or return characteristics. Thus, this paper examines whether any of these functions can be fulfilled by digital health stocks. **The general research question is how digital health is funded**, and to answer this question the author examines whether digital health stocks can be diversifiers or hedgers for the general market or alternative assets market to reduce risk or increase return in an investment portfolio. If so, this creates good prospects for future financing of digital health. If not, digital health financing may encounter problems.

Both primary and secondary **research methods** are used. Secondary research is conducted by way of analysis and comparison methods using various publications and practical reports with up-to-date data. Primary research is conducted by way of the author's own calculations, which include statistical methods.

DOI: 10.4324/9781032726557-5

The expected results contribute to the fragmentary and rare research on digital healthcare financing. More and more research is devoted to financing digital health (Kotenko & Bohnhardt, 2021; Kwon & Kim, 2022; Meessen, 2018), however this research does not show the investor's perspective, which influences the future of digital transformation. This chapter is unique, because apart from showing the recent years of development of venture capital and the strong and weak points of an IPO – the two most important ways of financing digital health, it aims to analyze perspectives and potential barriers to digital health transformation from the financial point of view.

Literature Overview

Digital health revolution needs financial support. Kotenko and Bohnhardt (2021) point out that the lack of funds in state budgets makes it difficult to improve and develop digital health services. Thus, it is obvious that money should come from other sources such as private funds like venture capital funds or should be gathered via stock exchanges. However, these methods of financing also involve certain obstacles, and it is a challenge to develop them. Also Safavi et al. (2020) pay attention to the problem of gathering funds for e-health development. The literature emphasizes the importance of early-stage funding for digital health (Adams, 2020), however if it is not continued in a public offer, the amount of funds is limited, as venture capital investors' funds are locked and cannot be used for other projects. Frimpong et al. (2022) analyze the influence of venture capital investments on the European health sector and find so many virtues that they advise more funding of this kind in this area. The authors also stress that funding prospects strongly depend on unforeseen situations such as the COVID-19 pandemic. For this reason, they conclude that it is important to encourage funding for the health sector. Simultaneously, as Zajicek and Meyers (2018) observe, apart from increasing the comfort of patients, digital health technologies finally decrease per capita costs, and thus they are worth developing not only from a social point of view but also from an economic one.

Digital health is broadly financed by venture capital and at a later stage this can be an IPO. According to Klonoff et al. (2019), digital health provides 10% of venture capital investments, which makes this field an important goal for the capital invested. Digital Health Business & Technology's (2021) data show that in 2014–2020, between four and seven companies went public in an IPO each year, and in 2021 this number rose suddenly to 20. Because of the fast development of digital health, further funds need to be gathered by attracting new investors. Simultaneously, funds supply is sensitive to the economic climate. According to Rock Health, US e-health funding increased from USD 1.6 billion in 2012 to USD 29.3 billion in 2021, however it sharply decreased in 2022 to USD 15.3 billion because of inflation, a bear stock market, and the risk of recession (Rock Health, 2023). This shows that the future of digital health depends also on the whole economy, and now the outlook is not optimistic.

Thus, gathering funds for such projects will probably be more difficult, and research on existing challenges, barriers, and perspectives is needed.

Venture capital financing is often followed by a public offering to help gather more funds and release the currently invested funds for early investors. This is because venture capital investors usually aim to engage their capital for a few years only (Cumming & Johan, 2010), and wish it to be released after this time. However, if investors are not interested in public issues, the venture has worse prospects for success. Thus, the crucial issue in determining barriers or perspectives of digital health financing is the role which digital equity can play in an investment portfolio. This is the issue examined by the author.

Factors Influencing Opportunities for Digital Health Companies to Raise Capital – The Strengths and Weaknesses of Venture Capital and IPO Financing in Digital Health

The chances of development of any start-up depend on financial support, and this can be provided by banks specializing in financing start-up. It has now become more difficult for digital health companies to acquire capital since the collapse of the Silicon Valley Bank in March 2023. It was an important institution providing capital to start-ups, and this included digital health. This shows that the overall economic situation may affect digital health companies' options for raising capital. The SVB went bankrupt due to becoming too dependent on the level of interest rates due to investing in treasury bonds. When interest rates rose, the price of bonds decreased and the need to sell bonds at lower prices led to its financial problems resulting in bankruptcy. Although for many years this bank's risk-based capital was higher than the banking industry average and American regulators considered it well-capitalized (Vo & Le, 2023), this approach resulted in disaster. Although digital health seems to have good prospects for development because of society's necessities, funding is not guaranteed.

The overall economic situation also affects the risk of a crash on the stock market. The higher the risk, the less likely investors are to decide to enter the digital health market. The economic situation risk also relates to private financing by venture capital. Investors are less eager to invest funds if the future of the economy is uncertain. From another point of view, the digital health sector may help investors diversify their investments. This sector should not be so sensitive to the general economic situation because healthcare is always needed, so there is always a demand for it. This rule can be applied to investors who lend their capital indirectly through a venture capital fund. Investors who only buy equity on stock markets are sensitive to speculative market fluctuations which, as the research conducted in this study shows, are even higher for the digital health sector, reflected by the S&P Kensho index, than for the S&P 500.

If companies want to be financed by venture capital, the ability to convince their managers to entrust the capital is very important. A successful track record in this or at least another field is important, as well as long-term contacts in the venture capital world.

The case of an initial public offering is different. It is not only a matter of convincing a venture capital fund but also the whole spectrum of market investors, to provide the capital. This is possible due to a good investment track record of earlier digital health companies listed on stock exchanges. Forecasting methods are based on historical returns (Chen et al., 2001), so if it is attractive, there are also encouraging prospects. If they have generated good results in the past, it is highly likely that potential investors will be more eager to risk their capital.

A venture capital company is a financial intermediary which gains capital from investors, seeks attractive investment opportunities, and engages in projects financed by the capital which it gathers (Gompers, 2001).

Figure 3.1 shows capital flows in a venture capital process. Stages 1 and 2 always occur, and stages 3 and 4 depend on the investment success and often do not occur.

As in the case of other financial intermediaries, one of the problems in venture capital investing is the information asymmetry between investors and institutions which need the capital. The latter are better acquainted with the market situation in the field in which they want to develop. This may lead to moral hazard (Krugman, 2009), which will mean that the entrepreneur may conceal some important information from investors. The less experienced the venture capital fund managers, the higher the risk of information asymmetry. It was first defined by Akerlof (1970) on the secondary market of cars, but this mechanism applies to financial markets as well. Du et al. (2020) show that this risk of information asymmetry may be mitigated if both parties have the same opinion regarding the investment environment. Glucksman (2020) points out that venture capitalists develop formal tools to reduce information asymmetry, unlike entrepreneurs, and this is their strength.

Advantages and disadvantages of venture capital financing can be analyzed from different points of view. The advantages for an investor are:

– reduction of both pre-investment and post-investment information asymmetry (Wynant et al., 2023);
– possibility of investing money in an alternative investment of low return, correlated with the market of traditional assets; and
– reduction of information asymmetry (Wynant et al., 2023).

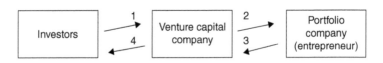

Figure 3.1 Directions and stages of capital flow in a venture capital process
Source: Author's study.

From an investor's point of view, the most important disadvantages are (Gompers & Lerner, 2001; Lerner & Tag, 2013, Lerner & Nanda, 2020):

- high risk that the financed company will not succeed, in other words there is no guarantee of profit or even to get the capital back;
- illiquidity of money invested – it is not possible to withdraw it before the period agreed in the earlier signed contract even if the return is unattractive; and
- returns are usually less regular than for traditional investments.

Advantages for an entrepreneur:

- It can gain funds to realize its business without the need to reveal business strategy and other important information to the public.
- It can be supported by a venture capitalist's knowledge and experience, which adds value (Sapienza, 1992).
- It has an opportunity to enhance its profitability through venture capital financing. (Kato and Germinah (2022) show that the general performance of VC financed companies is higher than those without VC.
- Venture capitalists play a crucial role in early-stage entrepreneur development due to providing competences such as screening, taking part in negotiations, or monitoring (Bonini & Capizzi, 2019).
- Tykvova (2007) points to the problem of the lack of managerial skills of an entrepreneur which seeks capital. The author emphasizes that thanks to the venture capital fund it may not only gather funds but also improve the management process and the goodwill of the company. This is achieved thanks to its specialization in a chosen field, which is stressed by Bengtsson and Bernhardt (2014). This helps to use the knowledge and managerial experience of the venture capital company,
- Some companies would not have a chance to develop without VC (Gompers, 2007).
- Venture capital increases innovation and the probability of success for its portfolio company (Bernstein et al., 2016).
- Proven positive influence on innovation (Faria & Barbosa, 2014).
- Positive impact on the economic growth of financed companies (Manigart & Sapienza, 2017).

The main disadvantages from the point of view of an entrepreneur seeking capital are:

- The venture capital company manages an investment together with an entrepreneur which in certain circumstances can be an advantage, however it may have a different opinion concerning directions of further development even if now of a transaction the opinions seem to be similar (Lerner & Tag, 2013).

- It may be time-consuming compared to an initial public offering or bond issue, as it requires establishing a relationship with a venture capitalist.
- It may be difficult to convince a venture capitalist to invest in some industries, and it requires establishing a long-term relationship (Glucksman, 2020).

As the data in Table 3.1 show, in 2011 the total transaction value was USD 1.2 billion and it increased to 29.1 in 2021. Apart from 2015, 2016, and 2019, the period 2011–2021 saw a rising trend on the digital health venture capital market. Unfortunately, in 2022 the total transaction value suddenly decreased by the highest value in the whole analyzed period (47.42%). The data for 2023 is for the first quarter only, however multiplying USD 3.4 billion by four gives a lower value (USD 13.6 million USD) than 15.3 for 2022. Therefore, the digital health venture capital market seems to have shrunk recently. This is also reflected by the number of transactions, which in 2022 for the first time decreased from 736 in the previous year to 575. For 2011–2021, the market increased gradually for the whole period. The average transaction value does not seem to reflect the market dynamics, because during the whole examined period, it fluctuated. In 2022, when the market collapsed it was still higher than at the beginning of the researched period.

Table 3.1 Venture capital invested in digital health in 2011–2023

Year	Number of Transactions[a]	Total Transaction Value (billion USD)	Annual Changes in Total Transaction Value (%)	Average Transaction Value (million USD)
2011	94	1.2		12.3
2012	146	1.6	33.33	10.8
2013	197	2.1	31.25	10.7
2014	298	5.4	157.14	15.2
2015	328	4.8	−11.11	14.7
2016	348	4.7	−2.08	13.5
2017	377	6.0	27.66	15.9
2018	395	8.6	43.33	21.7
2019	414	8.1	−5.81	19.6
2020	480	14.7	81.48	30.6
2021	736	29.1	97.96	39.5
2022	575	15.3	−47.42	26.6
2023[b]	132	3.4	−77.78	25.9

Source: Author's calculations and Rock Health Digital Health Venture Funding Database, https://rockhealth.com/insights/2023-q1-digital-health-funding-investing-like-its-2019/, access date: April 25, 2023.

[a] The data provider considers only transactions higher than 2 million USD.
[b] Data for 2023 are for the first quarter only.

In view of the above data, the digital health market may be encountering some problems with gathering funds in the form of venture capital. However, this may also mean that many digital health start-ups have been created over a period of more than a decade, and now it is time for market stabilization. If so, capital needs to be sought to release venture capital. An initial public offering can be a solution here.

A venture capitalist can engage its capital to conduct an initial public offering but also after some time of keeping funds invested, it may decide to go public. The possibilities of withdrawing funds through an IPO depend on historical data concerning raising capital in this way as well as historical data concerning risk and returns generated by equity issued by the digital sector. This issue is analyzed in one of the following parts of the chapter. The risk and returns of digital health sector equity are compared both with the general stock market and with some alternative assets.

An IPO is a process in which a company enters a public financial market by issuing stocks. It can be attractive for a venture capitalist to successfully exit an investment (Black & Gilson, 1998).

The research shows that even after an IPO, some companies decide to exit the public market. The main reasons they give for this are industry or market conditions and low price of their company assets. Moreover, managers usually analyze these factors from the point of view of the right time to enter a public market (Brau & Fawcett, 2006).

The downside of an IPO is that the research conducted in 1975–2020 shows that although the average return of IPO stocks is higher than for treasury bills, their median is lower (Huang et al., 2022). Such a conclusion means that only a small number of stocks generate attractive returns, whereas the majority do not perform better than treasury securities. Also Fang et al. (2021) prove that stocks do not perform better than treasury bills on international markets. The difference depends on the country, but the general rule is not favorable to stocks.

Literature enumerates the following among the main advantages of a company going public:

- reducing the cost of capital using outer capital (Modigliani & Miller, 1963);
- continual market valuation of a company, which tells managers whether it is correctly managed (Barden et al., 1984; Ghonyan, 2017);
- liquidity enabling new funds to be gathered if needed, also from venture capitalists, especially if a company shows good performance on a stock market (Barden et al., 1984; Ghonyan, 2017);
- possibilities of providing shares in a company or options to buy them at a favorable price to its managers to motivate them to develop it (Barden et al., 1984; Ghonyan, 2017);
- possibility of increasing the market share compared to competitors who do not decide to go public (Chemmanur & He, 2011);

- improved possibilities of raising additional funds in the future (Corman et al., 1989) as it strengthens the firm's credibility (Fahn et al., 2017);
- going public increases, the possibility of greater profitability (Larrain et al., 2021); and
- Brau et al. (2003) point out that an IPO helps to take over other companies.

The most important disadvantages of an IPO emphasized in scientific publications are:

- Necessity to cover costs of this process, which also include underpricing (Ritter, 1987) caused by information asymmetry between the internal and external environment (Lin, 2017). The reputation of an underwriter may help reduce the risk of underpricing in the short term (Carter et al., 1998). Costs are higher if an offering includes the underwriting process (Barry et al., 1991).
- Revealing all important information concerning the conducted activity to the public.
- Unlike debt financing, an IPO results in the dilution of capital, which means that capital lenders co-manage the company (Carbone et al., 2022).
- The risk of being underpriced, which is higher for developing stock markets, whereas the US stock market shows average returns for the first day at 16.8% (Teti & Montefusco, 2022).
- The risk of being taken over by another company (Brau et al., 2003).
- One of the factors which influence stock returns is information asymmetry, which is shown by Hutton et al. (2009). It also plays a role in the whole digital health sector financing process and makes these investments riskier both for investors lending their capital through venture capital, and for those which buy equity on the public stock market either in an IPO or on the secondary market. Myers and Majluf (1984) suggest that because of information asymmetry, financing by debt is better than by equity if external financing is required.

To sum up, the decision to go public depends on many factors such as the historical data, current market situation, the economic situation and its prospects, the sector in which a company operates, financial liquidity level, capital structure, and having other options regarding raising capital. An IPO may also be conducted when a venture capital fund wants to exit an investment. Venture capital has some advantages over an IPO, for example, not being obliged to make a company's situation public, or the possibility to use sophisticated knowledge and experience provided by a VC fund which can be a virtue for some entrepreneurs. Simultaneously, apart from some disadvantages, in many cases, VC may be the only opportunity for start-ups to start their business.

Methodology

In the first part of the research, the main descriptive statistics for analyzed assets are calculated. This is done following calculation of returns based on downloaded index values.

The following step is to verify whether digital health equity can be a portfolio hedger or diversifier for the general equity. This is done using Pearson correlation coefficient calculations in determined time periods.

Next the author checks the return and risk statistics of the S&P500 Total Return index (in USD) and the S&P Kensho Digital Health Total Return Index (in USD) to see if digital health stocks are worth investing compared to stocks in the main index in the context of the Markowitz (1952) theory. Next, the Kensho index is compared to some alternative assets like Bitcoin and crude oil. The launch date of S&P500 TR is March 4, 1957, and the first quotations date was January 3, 1928 (S&P 500, 2023), so the time for potential analysis is long. However, the research is limited to data available for S&P Kensho. The day of its first quotations was February 6, 2017, but hypothetical values are available from January 1, 2014 (S&P Kensho, 2023). Historical quotations of the index are given in Figure 3.2. Furthermore, S&P Kensho is compared to two alternative assets – Bitcoin (the main cryptocurrency) and crude oil.

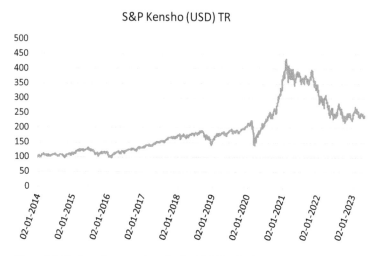

Figure 3.2 Stock market quotations for the S&P Kensho index from January 1, 2014 to May 11, 2023 (USD)

Source: Author's work based on data downloaded from: https://www.spglobal.com/spdji/en/indices/equity/sp-kensho-new-economies-composite-index/#overview, access date: 12.05.2023.

S&P Kensho is based on companies which provide remote healthcare services. It includes the following types of activities (S&P Kensho, 2023):

- remote monitoring of patients and patient diagnosis,
- platforms which provide or enable remote clinical services, surgeries, dentistry,
- solutions which the cloud to integrate medical data and their transfer,
- solutions enabling health administration in the cloud,
- platforms established to develop cooperation among medical professionals in treating patients, and
- platforms created to integrate healthcare providers with patients.

Therefore, the research period is from January 1, 2014 to May 11, 2023. This means that different periods can be considered in which there were extraordinary events such as the Covid-19 pandemic or Russia-Ukraine war, and different market trends, which makes conclusions more general. The analysis is conducted for different periods which depend on the trend observed on the market reflected by the S&P500 TR index. In particular, the following research periods are considered:

- January 1, 2014–February 19, 2020 – long-term rising trend on the stock market
- February 20, 2020–March 23, 2020 – declining trend caused by the COVID-19 pandemic
- March 24, 2020–January 3, 2022 – upward trend
- January 4 –October 12, 2022 – downward trend caused mainly by uncertainty resulting from the Russian-Ukrainian war
- October 13, 2022–May 11, 2023 – rising trend
- January 1–May 11, 2023 – the whole examined period which covers both stock market rises and decreases

The S&P 500 TR index is constituted of 500 companies quoted on the New York Stock Exchange and NASDAQ, which has the highest capitalization and covers about 80%. The Total Return Index also considers dividends which are paid out to investors (S&P Dow Jones, 2023). Its quotations for the research period are given in Figure 3.3.

For all assets, to achieve statistical measures, the first returns were calculated. Returns were also used together with risk to determine whether digital health sector assets can be diversifiers in an investment portfolio with traditional and alternative assets. As an association measure, the Pearson correlation coefficient was used.

This is mainly a standard deviation and is treated in this study as a risk measure. It is the second central moment of distribution and is calculated as a square root on variance of a single asset (Grobys, 2021), depending on the analyzed case. Additionally, skewness and kurtosis were applied (the third and the fourth central moments of the distribution).

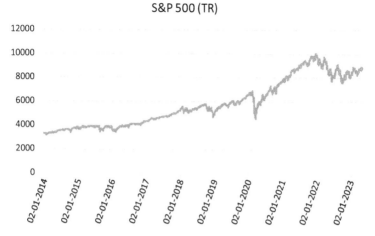

Figure 3.3 Stock market quotations of the S&P500 Total Return index from January 1, 2014 to May 11, 2023 (USD)

Source: author's work based on data downloaded from: available at: https://www.spglobal.com/spdji/en/indices/equity/sp-500/#data, access date: 12.05.2023.

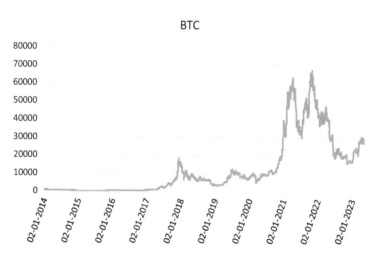

Figure 3.4 Daily prices of Bitcoin from January 1, 2014 to May 11, 2023 (USD)

Source: author's own study based on data downloaded from: https://stooq.pl/q/d/?s=btcusd&c=0&d1=20140101&d2=20230511, access date: 19.05.2023.

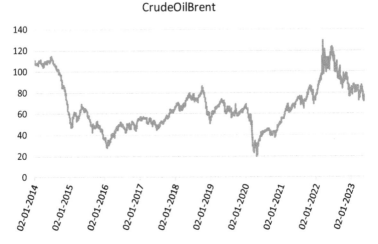

Figure 3.5 Daily prices of Brent crude oil from January 1, 2014 to May 11, 2023 (USD)

Source: author's work based on data downloaded from: https://stooq.com/q/?s=cb.c, access date: May 19, 2023.

Comparison of the Digital Health Sector with the General Equity Market and Alternative Assets

This part starts with the correlation analysis performed using Pearson correlation coefficients. Significance levels are presented beneath them. All underlined values are significant at 0.05.

As the data in Table 3.2 shows, correlation coefficients between returns on the S&P500 and S&P Kensho indexes are high (0.79 or higher) and significant (p = 0.0000) in each period. Correlations between S&P Kensho and Bitcoin are low, average, or insignificant. Correlations between S&P Kensho and crude oil are generally low or insignificant, except for the period February 20, 2020–March 23, 2020. Thus, the preliminary analysis of correlation coefficients suggests that digital health stocks cannot be diversifiers for traditional assets but can be portfolio diversifiers for alternative ones like crude oil or Bitcoin. It also shows that digital health stocks cannot be hedging assets for an investment portfolio because of positive correlation coefficients both with the traditional market and with the alternative one.

To answer the research question, it is necessary to calculate the main statistics of the S&P Kensho index and other analyzed assets taken for comparison. The results of the main statistics for S&P500 are given in Table 3.3.

From January 1, 2014 to February 19, 2020, the average return on S&P Kensho (0.037) was slightly lower than for S&P500 (0.042). S&P Kensho has also a standard deviation higher (1.48) than S&P500 (1.14). Both assets have a negative asymmetry of distribution, which is more negative for S&P (−0.81)

Table 3.2 Correlation table for analyzed assets

Correlation Table

January 1, 2014–February 19, 2020

	Crude oil	S&P500	SP Kensho	Bitcoin
Crude oil	1	0.19 (p=0.0000)	0.18 (p=0.0000)	−0.01 (p=0.8369)
S&P500	0.19 (p=0.0000)	1	0.89 (p=0.0000)	0.02 (p=0.5291)
SP Kensho	0.18 (p=0.0000)	0.89 (p=0.0000)	1	0.02 (p=0.3970)
Bitcoin	−0.01 (p=0.8369)	0.02 (p=0.5291)	0.02 (p=0.3970)	1

February 20, 2020–March 23, 2020

	Crude oil	S&P500	SP Kensho	Bitcoin
Crude oil	1	0.70 (p=0.0003)	0.78 (p=0.0000)	0.53 (p=0.0103)
S&P500	0.70 (p=0.0003)	1	0.96 (p=0.0000)	0.51 (p=0.0142)
SP Kensho	0.78 (p=0.0000)	0.96 (p=0.0000)	1	0.63 (p=0.0000)
Bitcoin	0.53 (p=0.0103)	0.51 (p=0.0142)	0.63 (p=0.0000)	1

March 24, 2020–January 3, 2022

	Crude oil	S&P500	SP Kensho	Bitcoin
Crude oil	1	0.26 (p=0.0000)	0.20 (p=0.0000)	0.12 (p=0.0114)
S&P500	0.26 (p=0.0000)	1	0.79 (p=0.0000)	0.25 (p=0.0000)
SP Kensho	0.20 (p=0.0000)	0.79 (p=0.0000)	1	0.31 (p=0.0000)
Bitcoin	0.12 (p=0.0114)	0.25 (p=0.0000)	0.31 (p=0.0000)	1

January 4, 2022–October 12, 2022

	Crude oil	S&P500	SP Kensho	Bitcoin
Crude oil	1	−0.0038 (p=0.9589)	0.01 (p=0.8589)	0.12 (p=0.0909)
S&P500	−0.0038 (p=0.9589)	1	0.90 (p=0.0000)	0.62 (p=0.0000)
SP Kensho	0.01 (p=0.8589)	0.90 (p=0.0000)	1	0.64 (p=0.0000)
Bitcoin	0.12 (p=0.0909)	0.62 (p=0.0000)	0.64 (p=0.0000)	1

(Continued)

Table 3.2 (Continued)

Correlation Table			
October 13, 2022–May 11, 2023			
	Crude oil	S&P500	SP Kensho	Bitcoin

	Crude oil	S&P500	SP Kensho	Bitcoin
Crude oil	1	0.31 (p=0.0002)	0.25 (p=0.0030)	0.05 (p=0.5193)
S&P500	0.31 (p=0.0002)	1	0.91 (p=0.0000)	0.35 (p=0.0000)
SP Kensho	0.25 (p=0.0030)	0.91 (p=0.0000)	1	0.40 (p=0.0000)
Bitcoin	0.05 (p=0.5193)	0.35 (p=0.0000)	0.40 (p=0.0000)	1

Source: Author's calculations.

Table 3.3 Descriptive statistics of logarithmic returns on the S&P500 TR Index from January 1, 2014 to May 11, 2023

Percentiles		Minimum values
1%	−3.39	−12.76
5%	−1.75	−9.97
10%	−1.11	−7.89
25%	−0.38	−6.06
50%	0.07	
		Maximum values
75%	0.56	6.06
90%	1.19	6.80
95%	1.59	8.91
99%	2.63	8.98
Number of observations	Mean	**Standard deviation**
2355	0.042	1.14
Variance	Skewness	Kurtosis
1.31	−0.81	18.79
Covariance with S&P Kensho	Correlation with S&P Kensho	
1.51	0.88 (p=0.0000)	

Source: Author's calculations.

than for S&P Kensho (−0.69). This means that negative returns are more probable for both assets than for standard normal distribution, and more probable for S&P 500 than for S&P Kensho. Kurtosis is higher for S&P 500 (18.79) than for S&P Kensho (10.12). Thus S&P500 returns are more heavy-tailed. To sum up, risk measures show different conclusions. The standard deviation suggests a lower risk level for the S&P 500, whereas the skewness and kurtosis are higher. Minimum values for all listed percentiles are lower for S&P Kensho than for the S&P500, which also shows that it is higher. In two cases, the maximum levels are higher for S&P Kensho, but for a 75% percentile the difference is very small (6.07 versus 6.06). To sum up, although the standard deviation and minimum percentile level show that the S&P Kensho index is a riskier investment, skewness and kurtosis show the opposite conclusion. Average returns are similar, so digital health stocks can be a desired asset for some investors interested in the development of this field. Also, because of high volatility, it may be a good idea to include it in a short-term speculative portfolio. From this point of view, they are rather not desired by long-term investors.

Moving on to the comparison of S&P Kensho with alternative assets, analysis of the data gathered in Tables 3.4 and 3.5 shows that in the period 2014–2023 risk measured with standard deviation was almost three times lower for the S&P Kensho index (1.48) than for Bitcoin (4.37). At the same time, Kensho skewness was negative and lower (−0.69 versus −0.23) and kurtosis higher (10.12 vs 8.06). Both measures show a higher risk level for digital health equity than for Bitcoin. The mean is lower (−0.04) versus (1.44), so the results do not encourage investors to entrust their funds to the digital health sector if they are innovative enough to invest in cryptoassets.

Comparison of the Kensho index with another alternative asset – crude oil – from January 2014 to May 2023 gives the opposite results. The mean for the Kensho index is positive (0.04) while the mean for crude oil is negative (−0.16). Simultaneously, all risk measures show that crude oil risk is higher than for the Kensho index. In particular, standard deviation is much lower for the Kensho index (1.48) than for crude oil (2.55). Skewness is much higher for Kensho (−0.69 and −1.22). Kurtosis is much lower for the Kensho index (10.12 versus 24.76). To sum up, statistical data shows that digital health industry investing may be a better option than crude oil – one of typical alternative assets.

Table 3.4 Descriptive statistics of logarithmic returns on the S&P500 TR Kensho Index from January 1, 2014 to May 11, 2023

Percentiles		Minimum values
1%	−3.96	−13.32
5%	−2.46	−11.37
10%	−1.70	−8.97
25%	−0.64	−8.50
50%	0.11	
		Maximum values
75%	0.83	6.07
90%	1.61	6.30
95%	2.16	7.40
99%	3.57	9.43
Number of observations	**Mean**	**Standard deviation**
2355	0.037	1.48
Variance	**Skewness**	**Kurtosis**
2.20	−0.69	10.12

Source: Author's calculations.

Table 3.5 Descriptive statistics of logarithmic returns on Bitcoin from January 1, 2014 to May 1, 2023

Percentiles		Minimum Values
1%	−12.79	−32.36
5%	−6.98	−24.02
10%	−4.38	−22.92
25%	−1.56	−22.55
50%	0.13	
		Maximum values
75%	2.01	19.34
90%	4.77	19.59
95%	7.27	19.76
99%	12.56	23.23
Number of observations	**Mean**	**Standard deviation**
2421	0.14	4.37
Variance	**Skewness**	**Kurtosis**
19.07	−0.23	8.06
Covariance with S&P Kensho	**Correlation with S&P Kensho**	
1.50	0.22	
	(p=0.0000)	

Source: Author's calculations.

Table 3.6 Descriptive statistics of logarithmic returns on Brent crude oil from January 1, 2014 to May 11, 2023

Percentiles		Minimum values
1%	−6.99	−30.74
5%	−3.84	−28.92
10%	−2.61	−16.06
25%	−1.03	−15.28
50%		
		Maximum values
75%	1.11	13.64
90%	2.39	14.61
95%	3.29	16.09
99%	6.53	19.08
Number of observations	**Mean**	**Standard deviation**
2341	−0.02	2.55
Variance	**Skewness**	**Kurtosis**
6.51	−1.22	24.76
Covariance	**Correlation with S&P Kensho**	
0.96	0.25	
	(p=0.0000)	

Source: Author's calculations.

Further analysis concentrates on comparisons of risk and return measures in different subperiods for S&P Kensho and alternative assets.

As the data gathered in Tables 3.7 and 3.8 show, correlations between returns on the S&P500 and S&P Kensho indexes are high (0.79 or higher) and significant (p = 0.0000) in each period. This means that the Kensho index

Table 3.7 Main statistics of logarithmic returns on the S&P500 TR Index from January 1, 2014 to May 11, 2023 divided into subperiods

January 1, 2014–February 19, 2020	Number of Observations	Mean	Standard Deviation	Variance
	1542	0.05	0.82	0.68
	Covariance	Correlation with S&P Kensho	Skewness	Kurtosis
	0.77	0.89 (p=0.0000)	−0.53	6.67
February 20, 2020–March 23, 2020	Number of observations	Mean	Standard deviation	Variance
	23	−1.79	5.10	26.03
	Covariance	Correlation with S&P Kensho	Skewness	Kurtosis
	25.42	0.96 (p = 0.0000)	0.07	2.94
March 24, 2020–January 3, 2022	Number of observations	Mean	Standard deviation	Variance
	450	0.17	1.25	1.56
	Covariance	Correlation with S&P Kensho	Skewness	Kurtosis
	1.85	0.79 (p=0.0000)	0.69	12.28
January 4, 2022–October 12, 2022	Number of observations	Mean	Standard deviation	Variance
	195	−0.14	1.52	2.32
	Covariance	Correlation with S&P Kensho	Skewness	Kurtosis
	2.89	0.90 (p=0.0000)	−0.22	2.94
October 13, 2022–May 11, 2023	Number of observations	Mean	Standard deviation	Variance
	145	0.106	1.21	1.47
	Covariance	Correlation with S&P Kensho	Skewness	Kurtosis
	1.74	0.91 (p=0.0000)	0.61	4.62

Source: Author's calculations.

cannot be a hedging or diversifying asset for general stock investments made by investors operating on the American stock exchange. In all the periods, standard deviations and variances are higher for S&P Kensho than for the S&P500, which means that risk understood as in the Markowitz theory is higher for the digital health sector than for stocks in general reflected by the S&P500, and the means are lower, with only one exception.

Table 3.8 Main statistics of logarithmic returns on the S&P Kensho TR Index from January 1, 2014 to May 11, 2023 divided into subperiods

January 1, 2014– February 19, 2020	Number of Observations	Mean	Standard Deviation	Variance
	1542	0.05	1.05	1.11
	Covariance	Correlation with S&P 500	Skewness	Kurtosis
	0.77	0.89 (p=0.0000)	−0.54	4.70
February 20, 2020– March 23, 2020	Number of observations	Mean	Standard deviation	Variance
	23	−2.062	5.17	26.71
	Covariance	Correlation with S&P 500	Skewness	Kurtosis
	25.42	0.96 (p = 0.0000)	−0.39	2.67
March 24, 2020– January 3, 2022	Number of observations	Mean	Standard deviation	Variance
	450	0.20	1.86	3.47
	Covariance	Correlation with S&P 500	Skewness	Kurtosis
	1.85661	0.79 (p=0.0000)	0.10	5.23
January 4, 2022– October 12, 2022	Number of observations	Mean	Standard deviation	Variance
	195	−0.22	2.09	4.39
	Covariance	Correlation with S&P 500	Skewness	Kurtosis
	2.89	0.90 (p=0.0000)	0.07	2.52
October 13, 2022– May 11, 2023	Number of observations	Mean	Standard deviation	Variance
	145	0.05	1.57	2.46
	Covariance	Correlation with S&P 500	Skewness	Kurtosis
	1.74	0.91 (p=0.0000)	0.21	3.25

Source: Author's calculations.

From January 2014 to February 2020, the S&P500 mean was 0.048, and for S&P Kensho it was 0.052 which means that it is slightly higher. Standard deviation is also higher (1.05 and 0.82) but only slightly. According to these measures, digital health stocks in this period were a better investment for investors with a higher risk tolerance. Skewness values are quite similar for both indexes (−0.53 for S&P500 and −0.54 for Kensho), whereas kurtosis shows that risk is lower for S&P Kensho (4.70) than for S&P500 (6.67).

In the next researched period, February 2020–March 2020, the S&P 500 mean was higher than for the Kensho index (−1.79; −2.06), however both are negative. Simultaneously S&P500 has a slightly lower standard deviation (5.10 and 5.17), so no investor would put its capital in digital health when the analysis is only made in the Markowitz environment. Also, skewness indicates that S&P Kensho is a worse selection due to negative skewness (−0.39) which means that negative returns are more probable than for the standard normal distribution, unlike the S&P500, where skewness is slightly positive (0.075). Kurtosis is lower for the S&P Kensho index (2.67) than for the S&P 500 (2.94), which shows that the former has a lower risk level.

From March 2020 to January 2022, the mean was slightly higher for S&P Kensho (0.20) than for the S&P 500 (0.18). The standard deviation is also higher for Kensho (1.86 versus 1.25), so the digital health sector is suitable for risk tolerant investors. Skewness shows that Kensho (0.098) is a worse investment than the S&P 500 (0.69) if only this measure is considered. Kurtosis shows the opposite. Kensho has a lower risk level (5.23) compared to the S&P 500 (12.28).

The next period, January 2022–October 2022, shows that both indexes have negative means, but for S&P Kensho it is more negative (−0.23 versus −0.14). As, in addition, the standard deviation is also higher for the same index, in this period digital health stocks were a worse choice than the general market. The opposite is true for skewness and kurtosis. The former is negative for the S&P 500 (−0.22) and slightly positive for Kensho (0.07). The latter is lower for Kensho (2.94 and 2.52), so both measures indicate a lower risk of loss.

The last research period, January 2014–May 2023, suggests that the S&P Kensho index generated a lower mean (0.05 versus 0.01) and a higher standard deviation (1.57 and 1.21), so a rational investor would not invest in it. The same is shown by skewness, which is lower for the S&P Kensho index (0.21 versus 0.61). Only kurtosis shows a lower risk level for the S&P Kensho index (3.25 versus 4.62).

The data in Tables 3.8 and 3.9 show that for all the created subperiods, the standard deviation of returns on the S&P Kensho index is lower than for Bitcoin. However, the former has also lower means for almost all periods (the exception is January–October 2022, but it is negative anyway). Thus, from the perspective of the Markowitz theory, the S&P Kensho index could be chosen by a risk-averse investor who considers either this cryptocurrency or the digital health sector as the target. Skewness and kurtosis show different results in different periods, often leading to contradictory conclusions on risk to standard deviations. For the period 2014–2020, the correlation coefficient between returns on Kensho and Bitcoin is low and insignificant, so the digital health sector could be a diversifier during this time. For other periods, correlation coefficients are average, so some investors could also consider digital health stocks in an alternative investment portfolio.

As the data in Tables 3.8 and 3.10 suggest, the Kensho index means are higher than for crude oil, except from January to October 2022. Standard deviations are lower in all subperiods for the Kensho index, which means that a

Table 3.9 Main statistics of logarithmic returns on Bitcoin from January 1, 2014 to May 11, 2023 divided into subperiods

January 1, 2014–February 19, 2020	Number of Observations	Mean	Standard Deviation	Variance
	1845	0.23	4.47	20.01
	Covariance with S&P Kensho	Correlation with S&P Kensho	Skewness	Kurtosis
	0.11	0.02 (p=0.3970)	−0.22	8.29
February 20, 2020–March 23, 2020	Number of observations	Mean	Standard deviation	Variance
	22	−1.81	9.44	89.08
	Covariance with S&P Kensho	Correlation with S&P Kensho	Skewness	Kurtosis
	31.50	0.63 (p=0.0000)	−1.30	6.54
March 24, 2020–January 3, 2022	Number of observations	Mean	Standard deviation	Variance
	460	0.42	4.19	17.54
	Covariance with S&P Kensho	Correlation with S&P Kensho	Skewness	Kurtosis
	2.36	0.31 (p=0.0000)	0.02	5.02
January 4, 2022–October 12, 2022	Number of observations	Mean	Standard deviation	Variance
	222	−0.46	4.19	17.54
	Covariance with S&P Kensho	Correlation with S&P Kensho	Skewness	Kurtosis
	5.63	0.64 (p=0.0000)	−0.84	7.30
October 13, 2022–May 11, 2023	Number of observations	Mean	Standard deviation	Variance
	149	0.22	3.49	12.16
	Covariance with S&P Kensho	Correlation with S&P Kensho	Skewness	Kurtosis
	2.24	0.40 (p=0.0000)	0.78	10.78

Source: Author's calculations.

rational investor in a Markowitz environment would choose the digital health sector out of these two possibilities. The risk measured with skewness and kurtosis shows different results in different periods.

The Kensho index can be a portfolio diversifier for crude oil investments in almost all the analyzed periods. Only during COVID-19, when all analyzed

Table 3.10 Main statistics of logarithmic returns on crude oil from January 1, 2014 to May 11, 2023 divided into subperiods

January 1, 2014– February 19, 2020	Number of Observations	Mean	Standard Deviation	Variance
	1524	−0.04	1.93	3.73
	Covariance with S&P Kensho	Correlation with S&P Kensho	Skewness	Kurtosis
	0.37	0.18 (p=0.0000)	0.26	7.93
February 20, 2020– March 23, 2020	Number of observations	Mean	Standard deviation	Variance
	22	−3.47	9.30	86.54
	Covariance with S&P Kensho	Correlation with S&P Kensho	Skewness	Kurtosis
	38.29	0.78 (p=0.0000)	−0.89	4.88
March 24, 2020– January 3, 2022	Number of observations	Mean	Standard deviation	Variance
	446	0.23	3.25	10.56
	Covariance with S&P Kensho	Correlation with S&P Kensho	Skewness	Kurtosis
	1.18	0.20 (p=0.0000)	−0.87	22.24
January 4, 2022– October 12, 2022	Number of observations	Mean	Standard deviation	Variance
	198	0.07	3.22	10.36
	Covariance with S&P Kensho	Correlation with S&P Kensho	Skewness	Kurtosis
	0.09	0.01 (p=0.8589)	−0.90	5.74
October 13, 2022– May 11, 2023	Number of observations	Mean	Standard deviation	Variance
	147	−0.15	2.16	4.67
	Covariance with S&P Kensho	Correlation with S&P Kensho	Skewness	Kurtosis
	0.84	0.25 (p=0.0030)	−0.04	2.85

Source: Author's calculations.

markets decreased, was the correlation coefficient between returns on Kensho and crude oil high. For all other periods, they were low, so these assets can be diversifiers for themselves, especially when one considers both returns and risk measures. However, they cannot be hedgers because of the positive correlation coefficients between these two groups of assets.

So, in short, taking the Markowitz model assumptions, investing in the digital health sector may be more attractive than investing in some alternative assets (crude oil) both from the point of view of risk measured with standard deviation and return. There is also a possibility of lower risk with a lower return for risk-averse investors compared to the cryptocurrency Bitcoin. The digital health sector can also be considered as a risk diversifier by alternative investment investors.

Final Findings and Limitations of the Study

As shown, an IPO and VC are totally different ways of financing the digital health sector and can provide different opportunities. However, they have a common feature, which is that investors must believe in success. This condition is more likely to be fulfilled if the general economic situation is good and stable.

If investors are not interested in public issues, venture capital has worse prospects for success. The comparison of statistics for analyzed assets shows that the digital health sector cannot be treated as a risk diversifier for the traditional American stock market. Correlations between returns on the S&P500 and S&P Kensho indexes are high (0.79 or higher) and significant ($p = 0.0000$) in each period. In all of the periods, standard deviations and variances are higher for S&P Kensho than for the S&P500, which means that risk understood as in the Markowitz theory is higher for the digital health sector than for stocks in general reflected by the S&P500. Means are mostly lower, so there is no reason to use digital health stocks as risk diversifiers in an investment portfolio. They cannot be applied to the hedging strategy either, as they are positively correlated with the traditional stock market.

The digital health sector has encountered some barriers with financing recently, and its future is not as bright as the past. One of the reasons for this may be that the novelty has worn off. Historical data shows that the digital health sector is not more attractive for investors than the general market reflected by the S&P500 index in the context of the Markowitz portfolio theory, which uses standard deviation as a risk measure. Other risk measures (skewness, kurtosis) show some advantages of the Kensho index over the S&P500, but only for some periods.

Different conclusions can be drawn on the diversifying role of the S&P Kensho index when it is compared to alternative assets such as Bitcoin or crude oil. In this context, it can be a diversifier for these alternative assets, especially for risk-averse investors. However, it does not perform better than the S&P500 index in the Markowitz theory context, so it is supposed to be rather used by industry investors who select this special sector for other reasons, for example, eagerness to choose good moments when this sector is supposed to grow more than the general market. As far as hedging is concerned, because of positive correlation coefficients, the digital health cannot play its role. In such a situation, digital health capital seekers should rather think about other ways of financing than entering a public market, such as venture capital, business angels, or own capital connected with some form of credit. Simultaneously, as an IPO is a popular method of exiting venture capital investments, it may also be difficult to gather capital using this method in the future.

As far as limitations of the study are concerned, additional commissions and costs of short selling are not considered in a similar way to the theory of classical finance (Markowitz, 1952). The analysis is conducted using the S&P 500 and S&P Kensho indexes. They reflect the general market situation of the companies which constitute them. If an investor buys or sells single stocks, the results may be different. Direct investments in indexes are not possible. Investors may use derivatives or invest in funds whose asset value is based on these indexes. In the case of CFD or futures contracts for S&P 500 application, the basis risk arises. The basis risk is understood as the difference between the price of a derivative and an underlying asset, which do not have to be equal. It can be measured with the correlation coefficient between a derivative and its underlying asset returns (Clement et al., 2018) and may influence the effectiveness of an investment.

These conclusions are important to all kinds of entrepreneurs, both individual and institutional. They may also be useful to digital health company managers as they show that some other ways of finding funds need to be found, based on the private market.

References

Adams, P. (2020). Financing your digital health venture. In S. Wulfovich & A. Meyers (Eds.), *Digital Health Entrepreneurship. Health Informatics* (pp. 59–70). Springer. https://doi.org/10.1007/978-3-030-12719-0_6

Akerlof, G. (1970). The market for lemons: Quality uncertainty and the market mechanism. *Quarterly Journal of Economics, 84*(3), 488–500. https://doi.org/10.2307/1879431

Barden, R. S, Copeland, J. E., Jr, Hermanson, R. H., & Wat, L. (1984, March). Going public-what it involves: A framework for providing advice to management. *Journal of Accountancy (pre-1986), 157*(000003), 63.

Barry, C. B., Muscarella, C. J., & Vetsuypens, M. R. (1991). Underwriter warrants, underwriter compensation, and the costs of going public. *Journal of Financial Economics, 29*(1), 113–135. https://doi.org/10.1016/0304-405X(91)90016-D

Bengtsson, O., & Bernhardt, D. (2014). Different problem, same solution: Contract specialization in venture capital. *Journal of Economics and Management Strategy, 23*(1), 396–426. https://doi.org/10.1111/jems.12055

Bernstein, S., Giroud, X., & Townsend, R. R. (2016). The impact of venture capital monitoring. *Journal of Finance, 71*(32), 1591–1622. https://doi.org/10.1111/jofi.12370.

Bitcoin. (2023). Data. Retrieved May 19, 2023, from https://stooq.pl/q/d/?s=btcusd&c=0&d1=20140101&d2=20230511

Black, B. S., & Gilson R. J. (1998). Venture capital and the structure of capital markets: Banks versus stock markets. *Journal of Financial Economics, 47*(3), 243–277. https://doi.org/10.1016/S0304-405X(97)00045-7

Bonini, S., & Capizzi, V. (2019). The role of venture capital in the emerging entrepreneurial finance ecosystem: Future threats and opportunities. *An International Journal of Entrepreneurial Finance, 21*(2–3), 137–175. https://doi.org/10.1080/1369106 6.2019.1608697

Brau, J. C., & Fawcett, S. E. (2006). Initial public offerings: An analysis of theory and practice. *The Journal of Finance, 61*(1), 399–436. https://doi.org/10.1111/j.1540-6261.2006.00840.x

Brau, J. C., Francis, B., & Kohers, N. (2003). The choice of IPO versus takeover: Empirical evidence. *Journal of Business, 76*(4), 583–612. https://doi.org/10.1086/377032

Carbone, E., Cirillo, A., Saggese, S., & Sarto, F. (2022). IPO in family business: A systematic review and directions for future research. *Journal of Family Business Strategy, 13*(3), 100433. https://doi.org/10.1016/j.jfbs.2021.100433

Carter, R., Dark, F., & Singh, A. K. (1998). Underwriter reputation, initial returns, and the long-run performance of IPO stocks. *The Journal of Finance, 53*(1), 28–311. https://doi.org/10.1111/0022-1082.104624

Chemmanur, T. J., & He, J. (2011). IPO waves, product market competition, and the going public decision: Theory and evidence. *Journal of Financial Economics, 101*(2), 382–412. https://doi.org/10.1016/j.jfineco.2011.03.009

Chen, J., Hong, H., & Stein, J. C. (2001). Forecasting crashes: Trading volume, past returns, and conditional skewness in stock prices. *Journal of Financial Economics, 61*(3), 345–381. https://doi.org/10.1016/S0304-405X(01)00066-6

Clement, K. Y., Botzen, W. J. W., Brouwer, R., & Aerts, J. C. J. H. (2018). A global review of the impact of basis risk on the functioning of and demand for index insurance. *International Journal of Disaster Risk Reduction, 28*(June), 845–853. https://doi.org/10.1016/j.ijdrr.2018.01.001

Corman, J., Perles, B., Catalan, A., & Bank, S. (1989). The initial public offering: a financing option for small businesses. *Journal of Business and Entrepreneurship, 1*(2), 81–94.

Crude Oil Brent Cash. (2023). Data. Retrieved May 19, 2023, from https://stooq.com/q/?s=cb.c

Cumming, D., & Johan, S. (2010). Venture capital investment duration. *Journal of Small Business Management, 48*(2), 228–257. https://doi.org/10.1111/j.1540-627X.2010.00293.x

Digital Health Funding and M&A Report – Q4 2021. (2021). *Digital Health Business & Technology.* https://digitalhealth.modernhealthcare.com/data-lists/digital-health-funding-and-ma-report-q4-2021, free version of cited data retrieved February 24, 2023, from https://digitalhealth.modernhealthcare.com/finance/after-record-breaking-2021-digital-health-ipos-are-nonexistent-2022

Du, P., Shu, H., & Xia, Z. (2020). The control strategies for information asymmetry problems among investing institutions, investors, and entrepreneurs in venture capital. *Frontiers in Psychology, 11*, 1–8. https://doi.org/10.3389/fpsyg.2020.01579

Fahn, M., Merlo, V., & Wamser, G. (2017). The commitment role of equity financing. *Working paper, 1712*, July, Department of Economics, Johannes Kepler University of Linz, Austria. Retrieved May 24, 2023, from http://www.econ.jku.at/papers/2017/wp1712.pdf

Fang, J., Marshall, B. R., Nguyen, N. H., & Visaltanachoti, N. (2021). Do stocks outperform treasury bills in international markets? *Finance Research Letters, 40*(C), 101710. https://doi.org/10.1016/j.frl.2020.101710

Faria, A. P., & Barbosa, N. (2014). Does venture capital really foster innovation? *Economics Letters, 122*(2), 129–131. https://doi.org/10.1016/j.econlet.2013.11.014.

Frimpong, F. A., Akwaa-Sekyi, E. K., & Saladrigues, R. (2022). Venture capital healthcare investments and health care sector growth: A panel data analysis of Europe. *Borsa Istanbul Review, 22*(2), 388–399. https://doi.org/10.1016/j.bir.2021.06.008

Ghonyan, L. (2017). Advantages and disadvantages of going public and becoming a listed company, June 29, available at SSRN. https://ssrn.com/abstract=2995271 or http://doi.org/10.2139/ssrn.2995271

Glucksman, S. (2020). Entrepreneurial experiences from venture capital funding: Exploring two-sided information asymmetry. *An International Journal of Entrepreneurial Finance, 22*(4), 331–354. https://doi.org/10.1080/13691066.2020.1827502

Gompers, P. (2007). Venture capital. In B. E. Eckbo (Ed.), *Handbook of Empirical Corporate Finance* (1st ed., pp. 481–509). Elsevier. https://doi.org/10.1016/B978-0-444-53265-7.50023-8

Gompers, P., & Lerner, J. (2001). The venture capital revolution. *Journal of Economic Perspectives, 15*(2), 145–168. https://doi.org/10.1257/jep.15.2.145

Grobys, K. (2021). What do we know about the second moment of financial markets? *International Review of Financial Analysis, 81*, 101891. https://doi.org/10.1016/j.irfa.2021.101891

Huang, G.-Ch., Liano, K., & Pan, M.-S. (2022). Do IPOs outperform treasury bills? *Finance Research Letters, 47*(A), 102610. https://doi.org/10.1016/j.frl.2021.102610

Hutton, A. P., Marcus, A. J., & Tehranian, H. (2009). Opaque financial reports, R2, and crash risk. *Journal of Financial Economics, 94*(1), 67–86. https://doi.org/10.1016/j.jfineco.2008.10.003

Kato, A. I., & Germinah, Ch.-P.E. (2022). Empirical examination of relationship between venture capital financing and profitability of portfolio companies in Uganda. *Journal of Innovation and Entrepreneurship, 11*(30), 1–18. https://doi.org/10.1186/s13731-022-00216-5

Klonoff, D. C., Evans, B., Zweig, M., Day, S., & Kerr, D. (2020). Is digital health for diabetes in an investment bubble? *Journal of Diabetes Science and Technology, 14*(1), 165–169. https://doi.org/10.1177/19322968198677

Kotenko, N., & Bohnhardt, V. (2021). Digital health projects financing: Challenges and opportunities. *Health Economics and Management Review ISSN (on-line), 1*, 100–107.

Krugman, P. (2009). *The Return of Depression Economics and the Crisis of 2008.* W.W. Norton.

Kwon, S., & Kim, E. (2022). Sustainable health financing for COVID-19 preparedness and response in Asia and the Pacific. *Asian Economic Policy Review, 17*(1), 140–156. https://doi.org/10.1111/aepr.12360

Lerner, J., & Nanda, R. (2020). Venture capital's role in financing innovation: What we know and how much we still need to learn. *Journal of Economic Perspectives, 34*(3), 237–261, https://doi.org/10.1257/jep.34.3.237

Lerner, J., & Tag, J. (2013). Institutions and venture capital. *Industrial and Corporate Change, 22*(1), 153–182. https://doi.org/10.1093/icc/dts050

Lin, Z. (2017). Background characteristics of Board Secretary and IPO Underpricing. *Modern Economy, 8*(11), 1340–1356. https://doi.org/10.4236/me.2017.811090

Lorrain, B., Philips, G. M., Sertsios, G., & Urzua, F. (2021). The effects of going public on firm performance and commercialization strategy: Evidence from international

IPOs. *NBER Working Paper Series. Working Paper 29219*. Retrieved May 24, 2023, from http://www.nber.org/papers/w29219; https://doi.org/10.3386/w29219

Maningart, S., & Sapienza, H. (2017). Venture capital and growth. In D. L. Sexton & H. Landstrom (Eds.), *The Blackwell Handbook of Entrepreneurship*. Wiley-Blackwell. https://doi.org/10.1002/9781405164214.ch12

Markowitz, H. (1952). Portfolio selection. *Journal of Finance, 7*(1), 77–91. https://doi.org/10.1111/j.1540-6261.1952.tb01525.x

Meessen, B. (2018). The role of digital strategies in financing health care for universal health coverage in low-and middle-income countries. *Global Health: Science and Practice, 6*(1), S29–S40.

Modigliani, F., & Miller, M. (1963). Corporate income taxes and the cost of capital: A correction. *American Economic Review, 53*(3), 433–443.

Myers, S. C., & Majluf, N. S. (1984). Corporate financing and investment decisions when firms have information that investors do not have. *Journal of Financial Economics, 13*(2), 187–221. https://doi.org/10.1016/0304-405X(84)90023-0

Ritter, J. R. (1987). The costs of going public. *Journal of Financial Economics, 19*(2), 269–281. https://doi.org/10.1016/0304-405X(87)90005-5

S&P 500 index. (2023). S&P Dow Jones Indices. (2023). Data. Retrieved May 12, 2023, from https://www.spglobal.com/spdji/en/indices/equity/sp-500/#data

S&P Dow Jones Index. (2023). S&P Dow Jones Indices. Retrieved May 8, 2023, from https://www.spglobal.com/spdji/en/indices/equity/sp-500/#overview

S&P Kensho Digital Health Index (2023). S&P Dow Jones Indices. Retrieved May 8, 2023, from https://www.spglobal.com/spdji/en/indices/equity/sp-kensho-digital-health-index-usd/#overview

S&P Kensho Digital Health Index. (2023). S&P Dow Jones Indices. Data. Retrieved May 12, 2023, from https://www.spglobal.com/spdji/en/indices/equity/sp-kensho-new-economies-composite-index/#overview

Safavi, K.C., Cohen, A. B., Ting, D. Y., Chaguturu, S., & Rowe, J. S. (2020). Health systems as venture capital investors in digital health: 2011–2019. *npj Digital Medicine, 3*(103), 1–5. https://doi.org/10.1038/s41746-020-00311-5

Sapienza, H. J. (1992). When do venture capitalists add value? *Journal of Business Venturing, 7*(1), 9–27. https://doi.org/10.1016/0883-9026(92)90032-M

Teti, E., & Montefusco, I. (2022). Corporate governance and IPO underpricing: Evidence from the Italian market. *Journal of Management and Governance, 26*(3), 851–889. https://doi.org/10.1007/s10997-021-09563-z

Tykvova, T. (2007). What do economists tell us about venture capital contracts. *Journal of Economic Surveys, 21*(1), 65–89. https://doi.org/10.1111/j.1467-6419.2007.00272.x.

Vo, L. V., & Le, H. T. T. (2023). From hero to zero – The case of Silicon Valley Bank, *Journal of Economics and Business* (forthcoming). http://doi.org/10.2139/ssrn.4394553

Wynant, L., Manigart, S., & Collewaert, V. (2023). How private equity-backed buyout contracts shape corporate governance. *Venture Capital, 25*(2), 135–160. https://doi.org/10.1080/13691066.2022.2109224

Zajicek, H., & Meyers, A. (2018). Digital health. In H. Rivas & K. Wac (Eds.), *Digital health. Scaling Healthcare to the World*. Springer.

2022 year-end digital health funding: Lessons at the end of a funding cycle. (2022). Retrieved February 24, 2023, from https://rockhealth.com/insights/2022-year-end-digital-health-funding-lessons-at-the-end-of-a-funding-cycle/

Part 2

Digitalization of Health Systems

Evidence from Poland

4 Digital Health in Poland

A Comparative Perspective

Julian Smółka and Martyna Smółka

Introduction: Digital Health and its Importance

Digital health is a significant topic for healthcare and its development (Desveaux et al., 2019). There is no single unified definition of this term, but Fatehi et al. (2020) analyzed more than 1,500 sources, both peer-reviewed and webpages. The one they provided will be used for this paper. Digital health is about the proper use of technology for improving the health and wellbeing of people at individual and population levels, as well as enhancing the care of patients through intelligent processing of clinical and genetic data.

In Web of Science for the topic "digital health," there are more than 40,000 published papers. When combined with "Poland," this leaves only 69. There are a number of reasons why digital health has become such a hot topic in recent years, and each of these reasons justifies the need to do research in this area in Poland.

Some of the reasons indicating how groundbreaking digital health can be for public health and healthcare systems are:

- Improved Access to Healthcare: technologies, such as telemedicine (Kruse et al., 2017) and mobile health apps, can significantly improve access to healthcare services, especially for individuals in remote or underserved areas.
- Enhanced Patient Engagement: tools like patient portals, wearable devices, and health apps allow patients to actively participate in their healthcare.
- Cost Efficiency: reducing healthcare costs by minimizing hospital visits and readmission rates, enabling early detection and management of health conditions, streamlining administrative tasks, and reducing the burden on healthcare staff (Gentili et al., 2022).
- Improved Quality of Care: enhancing the quality of care by enabling real-time monitoring of patients, personalized treatment plans, immediate response to medical emergencies, evidence-based decision-making, and improved coordination among healthcare providers (Lin et al., 2019).
- Data Collection and Research: vast amounts of health data can be used for research, disease surveillance, and public health initiatives, which can lead

DOI: 10.4324/9781032726557-7

to new insights, a better understanding of diseases, and the development of new treatments (Rieke et al., 2020).

- Health Equity: addressing health disparities by improving access to healthcare services among marginalized and underserved communities (Brewer et al., 2020).
- Response to Health Crises: maintaining healthcare services during lockdown, enabling remote patient monitoring, and facilitating contact tracing and dissemination of health information (Williams et al., 2022).

The study aims to determine the state of digital health in Poland and create a *Digital Health Profile* (DHP) – that summarizes information about the country's context, health priorities, advancements in digital health, and quality improvement efforts (Liaw et al., 2021, p. 495). To do this, we compare measurement tools and select one to use for a comprehensive analysis of Polish digital health. The results can serve as a basis for further research on the topic, devoted in detail to each of the outlined areas, but also as a guide for politicians, policymakers, and health economists interested in the field (Jandoo, 2020).

How to Analyze the State of Digital Health

Digital health maturity models are frameworks that help organizations assess their current level of digital health capabilities and guide them toward achieving higher levels of maturity. These models typically consist of multiple stages or levels, each representing a different degree of sophistication in the use of digital health technologies. These models can be used to identify gaps, set goals, and track progress over time. However, it is important to note that the journey toward digital health maturity is not linear and may vary greatly depending on the specific context and needs of each organization.

There are four popular models in literature for assessing the maturity of digital health (Liaw et al., 2021). Each of these models has a unique perspective and focus, providing a comprehensive understanding and assessment of digital health maturity across various aspects and levels of healthcare organizations. These are compared in Table 4.1.

For all the models, GDHI – dedicated to analyzing the state of digital health in individual countries – will best serve the purpose of our analysis. In our analysis, we use the entire model and do not subject it to any modifications, ensuring comparability with results for other countries.

Digital Health Index Methodology

The GDHM team, in collaboration with representatives from over 20 countries and more than 50 international agencies and organizations, developed

Table 4.1 Selected digital health maturity assessment models comparison

Maturity Assessment Models	Focus of Model	Maturity Categories	Maturity Descriptors
Informatics Capability Maturity Model (ICMM)	Health organization	– Managing information – Using business intelligence – Using information technology tools – Aligning business and informatics – Managing change	General descriptors with examples for five levels of maturity: basic, controlled, standardized, optimized, and innovative. Respondents reflect on their digital health profile and choose a maturity level.
Global Digital Health Index (GDHI)	National digital health system	– Leadership & Governance – Strategy & Investment – Legislation, Policy & Compliance – Workforce – Standards & Interoperability – Infrastructure – Services & Applications.	Prescriptive descriptors with respondent ticking one out of five specific statements for each category and subcategory ranked according to levels of maturity.
Health Information Systems Interoperability Maturity Toolkit (HISIMT)	Health organization (technical & operational)	– Leadership and governance – Human resources – Technology – There are several subcategories.	Prescriptive descriptors with respondent ticking "yes/no" for one out of five specific statements for each category and subcategory to ascertain five levels of maturity: nascent, emerging, established, institutionalized, or optimized.
Health Information System Stages of Continuous Improvement Toolkit (HISSCIT)	Health organization (technical & operational)	– Leadership & Governance – Management – ICT infrastructure – Systems – Interoperability – Data quality – Data use	Prescriptive with respondent ticking "yes/no" for one out of five specific statements for each category and subcategory to ascertain five levels of maturity: Emerging / Ad hoc, Repeatable, Defined, Managed, or Optimized.

Source: Liaw et al. (2021) A digital health profile & maturity assessment toolkit: cocreation and testing in the Pacific Islands, Journal of the American Medical Informatics Association.

the first version of the GDHI in early 2016. In 2022, the resource underwent a comprehensive review and redesign process that lasted a year. This process aimed to align the indicators with the WHO Global Digital Health Strategy, with an increased focus on AI, equity, gender, and Universal Health Coverage (UHC). The name was also changed to the GDHM to better reflect its role in tracking digital health progress at the country, regional, and global levels.

The GDHM team developed the indicators by conducting a global data landscape review available through multilateral organizations, mapping available data by reviewing existing frameworks and tools, and convening digital health experts to refine and define an initial set of recommended indicators into a manageable list.

Data for each country is collected in collaboration with country partners and Ministry of Health representatives leading digital health efforts in their respective countries. These partners submit their country's data through an annual GDHM survey, selecting the appropriate phase for each indicator and providing a rationale and evidence to support these phases. The GDHM team verifies the collected data before publishing it.

The GDHM uses the main indicators in each category to calculate the overall country average. Sub-indicators add greater specificity to specific GDHM indicators but are not used in calculating the Component Phase or the Country or Global Averages. The GDHM allows countries to benchmark themselves against the Global Average or a specific overall phase.

For countries that have not completed a survey in the GDHM, data was extracted from publicly available information to pre-populate certain indicators. This data serves as a proxy for these digital health indicators for countries, but data completed by government officials provide a more accurate and robust picture of the digital health progress in each country (Digital Health Monitor, 2023). Poland was one of the countries for which the data was pre-populated. In the indicators where it took place, we compare our results and assessment with the ones from the Digital Health Monitor.

The research conducted in this study aims to provide a comprehensive analysis of the state of digital health in Poland. To ensure a scientific approach, we used various research methods and techniques to develop an assessment. The study employed a methodological framework based on scoping review methodology, which allows a systematic and comprehensive analysis of existing literature and data.

The methodology utilized several techniques commonly used in social sciences research, including content analysis, document analysis, and literature searches. These methods enabled the researchers to gather relevant legal texts, reports, and publicly available data to assess the current state of digital health in Poland. One of the key aspects of the analysis was to examine legal acts and legislation, and digital health strategies that are being implemented at the national level. By employing these techniques, the study ensured a rigorous analysis of the subject matter.

Digital Health Index for Poland

Using the GDHM framework, we analyze the healthcare system in Poland in terms of its digital state in seven areas: (I) Leadership & Governance, (II) Strategy & Investment, (III) Legislation, Policy, and Compliance, (IV) Workforce, (V) Standards & Interoperability, (VI) Infrastructure, and (VII) Services and Applications. We assess the state of Poland's digital health development on a scale of 1–5 in each of 23 indicators (Mechael & Edelman, 2019).

Leadership & Governance

Poland has a well-established digital health governance structure that works and is led by the government. The Ministry of Health oversees e-Health development, with ongoing support from the e-Health Centre (CeZ). The CeZ actively manages the digital health sector, collaborating with ministries and vigilantly monitoring AI-based initiatives (e-Health Centre, 2023b).

Public entities are pivotal stakeholders in the CeZ's solution implementation, serving as business owners and as members on project steering committees. Key stakeholders, including the Ministry of Health, the National Health Fund, National Blood Center, Main Pharmaceutical Inspectorate, Main Sanitary Inspectorate, and medical universities, actively contribute to shaping e-health policy (e-Health Centre, 2023a).

The "e-Health Centre Strategy 2023–2027" reveals a proactive governance structure, monitoring digital health, and data governance implementation, including integration of AI technologies. The mention of a work plan further indicates the structured approach to governing digital health initiatives. The strategy highlights the importance of AI in e-Health and acknowledges the rapid development of AI-based technology. It mentions the need to strengthen resources in the area of AI and the creation of a specialized AI team within the e-Health Centre (e-Health Centre, 2023a). In 2020, the Policy for the Development of AI in Poland was approved, which also addresses the use of AI in healthcare and the challenges behind its use (Resolution no. 196 of the Council of Ministers of December 28, 2020).

Referring back to the "e-Health Centre Strategy 2023–2027," the document acknowledges the significance of digital health, addressing benefits and risks. It emphasizes cybersecurity measures, including competence enhancement, information sharing, and rapid response to threats, ensuring e-Health system security and minimizing risks to public health and individuals (e-Health Centre, 2023a). While strategies for various considerations are outlined, some may still be in the process of implementation.

The e-Health Development Programme is an operational and implementation document that aims to implement public policy in the area of digital health. The program primarily refers to the Ministry of Health's strategic document "Healthy Future. Strategic framework for the development of the healthcare system for 2021–2027, with an outlook to 2030" (Healthy Future) and focuses on its main conclusions and set goals. The main areas of the program include greater patient involvement in their own health, patient health prediction and decision support, deinstitutionalization and care coordination, communication and consultation, and pharmacotherapy support. The program also aims to develop telemedicine tools, improve care coordination, and develop electronic medical records. The e-Health Development Programme also fits more broadly into the strategy of the Polish healthcare system. It references other national documents, such as the "National Plan for Reconstruction and Increasing Resilience" and the "Polish New Deal." An important aspect of the program is the development of digital competencies for patients, medical personnel and other health professions, and the development of ICT systems and medical records. The program aims to improve the quality, accessibility, and openness of medical data and to ensure coordination of activities and cooperation among various participants in the healthcare system (Ministry of Health, 2022a, pp. 3–9). The Program (Ministry of Health, 2022a, p. 22) includes educational activities to minimize inequalities in access to digital health services (e-Health Centre, 2023a; Resolution of the Council of Ministers of March 30, 2021). The documents described show that consideration of new technologies is evident in both the country's overall health strategy (Ministry of Health, 2021a) and area strategy documents (e-Health Centre, 2023a; Ministry of Health, 2022a). The need to increase their use and directions for development in systemic healthcare is indicated.

The country recognizes the importance of digital health and has incorporated and implemented it into its strategic planning framework, which is being periodically evaluated and optimized. However, area documents are not updated, and information on their progress is not released to the public. Measures of their success have not been formulated.

Challenges in the areas of diversity, equality, and human rights have been identified and analyzed in the Strategic Framework for Health Care in Poland (Ministry of Health, 2021a) and are addressed directly in the strategic and operational objectives specified in the National Health Programme (Ministry of Health, 2021b). The funding for particular initiatives is divided through the National Health Programme. The implementation of the particular e-health initiatives is led by the CeZ.

The Strategic Framework for Health Care in Poland addresses gender issues and health inequalities (Ministry of Health, 2021a, pp. 5–17). Lack of planned activities specifically affects the transformation of gender roles and relations in the healthcare system (Table 4.2).

Strategy & Investment

Poland has taken significant steps in advancing its digital health sector by approving a national digital health cost plan. The e-Health Centre is a state budget unit under the authority of the minister responsible for healthcare

Table 4.2 Results summary concerning Leadership & Governance category in Polish digital health

Indicator No.	Indicator Description	Score	Score Description
1	Digital health prioritized at the national level through dedicated bodies / mechanisms for governance	4	Governance structure is fully functional, government-led, consults with other ministries, and monitors implementation of digital health and data governance, including artificial intelligence, based on a work plan.
2	Digital Health prioritized at the national level through planning	5	Digital health is implemented and periodically evaluated and optimized in national health or other relevant national strategies and/or plans.
2a	Health is prioritized in national digital transformation and data governance policies	4	National digital transformation and data governance policies systematically include potential benefits and risks for public health or individual health outcomes and have some strategy(ies) for addressing them that are not yet implemented.
3	Readiness for emerging technologies adoption and governance	4	A plan for one or more emerging technologies (e.g., AI, Wearables, Blockchain, IoT) to support public health is being implemented, is funded, and the results are being monitored. Governance mechanisms required for emerging technologies are in place.
4	Diversity, Equity, and human rights analysis, planning and monitoring included in national digital health strategies and plans	5	Poland is implementing and evaluating the effects of digital health strategies and specific digital health solutions based on equity and human rights impact assessments. Documented strategies are in place to address gaps in access and outcomes for different population groups, including women, children, and marginalized groups.
4a	Gender considerations accounted for in digital health strategies and digital health governance	3	Digital health strategies and programs are developed and implemented with systematic consideration of gender norms, roles, and relations without the policies or structures for accountability (gender-sensitive).

Source: Authors' work based on the Digital Health Monitor.

information systems (Order of the Minister of Health of June 4, 2020). The plan sets the strategic direction and priorities for the country's digital health initiatives, including a thorough assessment of associated costs (e-Health Centre, 2023a). Despite the establishment of a structured state budget line item for the e-Health Centre's operations and the implementation of the e-Health Development Programme, there is a recognition that the allocated funding may be moderately insufficient. To fully address digital health priorities and ensure effective implementation, additional financial resources may be required (Ministry of Health, 2022a, p. 8; e-Health Centre, 2023a).

Poland's "e-Health Centre Strategy 2023–2027" outlines a comprehensive strategy for the development of digital health in Poland, which is aligned with the principles of UHC (WHO, 2023). The strategy focuses strongly on the integration of digital health services, the enhancement of data-driven decision-making processes, and the establishment of a competent digital health center (e-Health Centre, 2023a).

The strategy addresses several core UHC components, including coverage, access, uptake, quality, and equity. The strategy does not, however, explicitly mention the inclusion of metrics to assess the contribution of digital health toward UHC goals. Therefore, the ultimate score of the indicator was lowered. The document includes specific goals related to the improvement of internal processes and the development of key competencies.

Poland has achieved UFC with more than 90% coverage of the population with an affordable basic set of services. In the category of depth of coverage (prepayment schemes) for health services, Poland scored 96%, 73%, 33%, and 65%, respectively, for Inpatient Care, Outpatient Primary and Specialist Care, Pharmaceuticals, and Ancillary services (OECD, 2016).

The private sector actively engages in digital health activities, demonstrating a systematic approach to participation and investment in this sector. It is both self-organizing and undertakes digital health activities and investments (Pokrzycka-Walczak, 2023) and also collaborates with the public sector on common challenges (Zielonacki, 2019) and investments and works in dialogue with the academic community (Medycyna Prywatna, 2022). The current level of private sector participation and investment, however, may not fully meet the country's digital health needs (Table 4.3).

Legislation, Policy, & Compliance

Since May 25, 2018, the General Data Protection Regulation (GDPR) has been in force in all EU member states, including Poland (Regulation (EU) 2016/679). The GDPR provides a legal framework for data protection, including security and cybersecurity measures, and sets standards for the collection, processing, storage, transmission, use, and destruction of personal data, including health data, within the EU. The proposed score is based on the assessment that the GDPR may not be yet consistently applied, which is confirmed, for instance, by data published by the Office for Personal Data Protection (UODO) (Sanocki, 2021). The inconsistent implementation is demonstrated by the reported GDPR violations and filed official complaints filed with the UODO.

Table 4.3 Results summary in the area concerning Strategy & Investment category in Polish digital health

Indicator No.	Indicator Description	Score	Score Description
5	National e-Health/ Digital Health Strategy or Framework	3	National digital health costed plan developed and approved.
5a	National digital strategy alignment with UHC Core Components	4	Digital health strategy exists and is fully aligned with the country's UHC goals, but does not include metrics to assess the contribution of digital health toward UHC goals.
6	Public funding for digital health	4	A structured and systematic budget line item for digital health exists but is moderately insufficient (above 50% of the need) to meet the country's digital health needs.
6a	Private sector participation and investments in digital health	3	The private sector participation and investment in the country's digital health activities is systematic but does not meet the needs of the country.

Source: Authors' work based on Digital Health Monitor.

The Act on the Protection of Personal Data applies in Poland and provides regulations for the protection of individual privacy, including ownership, consent, access, and sharing of individually identifiable health data, including digital health data (The Act of May 10, 2018, on the Protection of Personal Data). Additionally, the Act on the Protection of Health Information and Medical Documentation addresses confidentiality and access to health information (The Act of April 28, 2011, on the Information System in Health Care). While these laws exist, have already been implemented, and contain the necessary provisions for privacy protection, there may be variations in their implementation and enforcement across different contexts or entities within the healthcare system. Hence, a score of four was given to reflect the inconsistency in enforcement.

The e-Health Development Programme (Ministry of Health, 2022a) defines the state of affairs and the necessary actions to be taken in shaping policies, protocols, and frameworks, regarding telemedicine, AI, and management of data generated using the latest technologies. The precepts of the program are being systematically implemented, as reflected in the CeZ Development Strategy (e-Health Centre, 2023a).

As part of the Ministry of Health's POPI Investment Project Support Platform, it is possible to certify health mobile applications in terms of technical requirements, security level, and patient privacy (Ministry of Health, 2023).

The Act on Medical Devices provides regulations and requirements for the use of medical devices (The Act of April 7, 2022, on Medical Devices).

Poland has a policy for the development of AI, which also includes the use of AI in healthcare systems (Resolution no. 196 of the Council of Ministers of December 28, 2020). Protocols, frameworks, or accepted processes governing AI use in healthcare services have been proposed and are under review on both the EU and national levels. There is still ongoing development and refinement needed to establish a comprehensive and fully implemented regulatory framework for AI in healthcare in Poland (European Parliament, 2023).

With regard to cross-border health data exchange and security, Poland is implementing the recommendations of the EU in this area and developing its own initiatives (Directive 2011/24/EU of the European Parliament and of the Council of March 9, 2011). A system of cross-border prescriptions has been created, allowing the filling in of Polish e-prescriptions in Croatia, Spain, and Finland, and the filling in of prescriptions in Poland written by doctors of the same countries as above and Estonia. The program is being further developed within the EU, and more countries are expected to be gradually included in the system (European Commission, 2023). In 2023, the e-Health Centre is also scheduled to launch electronic cross-border patient card solutions (Table 4.4).

Workforce

In Poland, the following medical professions are regulated by law: physician, dentist, pharmacist, nurse, midwife, laboratory diagnostician, physiotherapist, and paramedic. Standards of training for this profession are determined by a regulation of the Minister of Science and Higher Education. Digital health-related education is included only in the requirements for physicians and paramedics, and only at a very basic level (Regulation of the Minister of Science and Higher Education of July 26, 2019).

Digital health is not a part of the curriculum for health and health-related support professionals, and there are no public dedicated training programs or information on possible plans to open such educational paths. There are no strategy, defined career paths, or guides in the public sector for hiring and development of digital health professionals. The implemented activities do not include systemic education in digital health. The existing efforts are limited in scope and not widely implemented.

In early 2023, the Council of Ministers of the Republic of Poland adopted a resolution introducing the Digital Competence Development Programme. One of the envisaged measures is to strengthen digital competencies in healthcare, including the organization of personalized training in digital competencies, comprising modern medical technologies, e-health services, and cyber security (Resolution no. 24 of the Council of Ministers of February 21, 2023). The program outlines plans to train 1,000 individuals in e-health, telemedicine, the use of modern technologies in medicine, and cyber security

Table 4.4 Results summary concerning Legislation, Policy, & Compliance category in Polish digital health

Indicator No.	Indicator Description	Score	Score Description
7	Legal Framework for Data Protection (Security / Cybersecurity)	4	There is a law on data security (covering the full data lifecycle, e.g., collection, processing, storage, transmission, use and destruction), that is relevant to digital health that has been implemented, but not consistently enforced.
8	Laws or Regulations for privacy, consent, confidentiality and access to health information (Privacy)	4	There is a law to protect individual privacy, governing ownership, access, consent, and sharing of individually identifiable digital health data that has been implemented but not consistently enforced.
9	Protocol for regulating or certifying devices and/or health services- including provisions for AI and algorithms (at higher stages of maturity)	3	Protocols, policies, frameworks, or accepted processes governing the clinical and patient care use of connected medical devices and digital health services have been passed, but are not fully implemented.
9a	Protocol for regulating and certifying AI within health services	2	Protocols, policies, frameworks, or accepted processes governing AI use in healthcare have been proposed and are under review
10	Cross-border data security and sharing	3	Protocols, policies, frameworks or accepted processes for cross-border data exchange and storage in support of public health goals while protecting individual privacy have been passed, but are not fully implemented

Source: Authors' work based on the Digital Health Monitor.

(Resolution no. 24 of the Council of Ministers of February 21, 2023). There is, however, no publicly available information on the launch of the program. Previously, 1,648 medical specialists were trained in the project "Improving the quality of management in healthcare through the dissemination of ICT knowledge" (Neumann, 2015; Table 4.5).

Standards & Interoperability

An existing and functional architectural framework and health informa-tion exchange has been established. The CeZ architectural repository is a central source of truth for architectural and analytical knowledge in the area of digital health in the perspectives: business, applications, data, and

Table 4.5 Results summary concerning the Workforce category in Polish digital health

Indicator No.	Indicator Description	Score	Score Description
11	Digital health integrated in health and related professional pre-service training (prior to deployment)	3	Digital health curriculum implementation underway covering an estimated <50% of health professionals in pre-service training.
12	Digital health integrated in health and related professional in-service training (after deployment)	2	Digital health curriculum proposed and under review as part of in-service (continuing education) training for health professionals in the workforce.
13	Training of digital health workforce	1	There is no training available for the digital health workforce in the country.
14	Maturity of public sector digital health professional careers	1	No workforce strategy, policy, or guide that recognizes digital health is in place. Distribution of digital health workforce is ad hoc.

Source: Author's work based on Digital Health Monitor.

technology. The CeZ repository is based on Confluence environment, Prolaborate environment, and Enterprise Architect environment (EA repository). The architecture of all of the CeZ systems is migrated to a common CeZ analytical and architectural environment, and new systems are created and standards introduced to enable the acquisition/building, development, and deployment of IT solutions that will improve interoperability, minimize duplication, and simplify the IT environment in all areas of the CeZ. An architecture content metamodel was also created, defining the most essential architectural elements of the CeZ necessary for building interop e-government systems. The metamodel is based on TOGAF (The Open Group Architecture Framework), which delineates within enterprise architecture a comprehensive approach to the design, planning, implementation, and management of an organization's enterprise architecture. The CeZ architecture follows the principles developed as part of the State Information Architecture, which is the overarching architecture (e-Health Centre, 2023a, pp. 47–48).

One of the strategic goals of the e-Health Centre is to standardize e-health services. There is an Interoperability Council at the CeZ, which is an organization representing the main stakeholders (representatives of central offices, medical entities, patients, standardization organizations, and software manufacturers) and has an advisory and opinion-making role.

In its strategy, the CeZ points to the implementation of the data model standardization within the healthcare system, and to the development of the needed semantic interoperability for data structuring. The implementation and

Table 4.6 Results summary concerning Standards & Interoperability category in Polish digital health

Indicator No.	Indicator Description	Score	Score Description
15	National digital health architecture and/or health information exchange	5	Data standards are routinely updated and data is actively used for monitoring and evaluating the healthcare system and for national health strategic planning and budgeting.
16	Health information standards	2	There are some digital health / health information standards for data exchange, transmission, messaging, security, privacy, and hardware that have been adopted and/or are used.

Source: Authors' work based on the Digital Health Monitor.

application of SNOMED clinical terminology will enhance the interoperability of IT systems within healthcare, thereby paving the way for solutions based on AI. The terminology will be accessible in the Registry of Coding Systems (e-Health Centre, 2023a, pp. 50–51; Table 4.6).

Infrastructure

The Network Readiness Index (NRI) score for Poland is obtained from the Portulans Institute's Technology Pillar of the Network Readiness Index. Poland was awarded a score of 50.61 for network readiness, placing 44th. The assessment takes into account various factors related to access, content, and future technologies. While Poland performs well in certain aspects such as population coverage by at least a 3G mobile network and internet access in schools, there is room for improvement in areas like the adoption of emerging technologies and robot density (Portulans Institute, 2022).

The score of 50.61 has been rounded down, as of the three categories that make up the Technology pillar, only one is above 50. Poland achieved a score of 76.09 in the Access category, in which it ranked first in no less than two subcategories (Portulans Institute, 2022).

Infrastructure development in Poland is carried out in three strategic documents: Healthy Future (Ministry of Health, 2021a, pp. 97–112), setting the general directions in this regard, the e-Health Development Programme, indicating the areas and priorities for the development of digital health infrastructure, and the e-Health Centre Development Strategy (e-Health Centre, 2023a, pp. 47–48), indicating precisely what systems and solutions will be built and implemented in the CeZ itself, as the unit centrally responsible for the development of e-Health in Poland, and in the individual entities that make up the entire system.

Table 4.7 Results summary concerning Infrastructure category in Polish digital health

Indicator No.	Indicator Description	Score	Score Description
17	Network readiness	3	26–50
18	Planning and support for ongoing digital health infrastructure maintenance	4	A plan for supporting digital health infrastructure (including equipment- computers/ tablets/ phones, supplies, software, devices, etc.) provision and maintenance has been implemented partially and consistently with an estimated 25–50% of necessary digital health infrastructure needed in the public healthcare service sector available and in use.

Source: Authors' work based on the Digital Health Monitor.

As part of the implemented and planned activities, the construction of a coherent architecture of systems based on a private cloud with high availability is envisaged (e-Health Centre, 2023a, pp. 47–48).

Infrastructural changes in the healthcare system, including the adaptation of infrastructure to digital health services, are also envisaged in the National Reform Programme and are to be implemented in large part with funds under the National Recovery Plan (KPO) (National Reform Programme 2023/2024, 2023, p. 61; Table 4.7).

Services & Applications

Poland has implemented scaled digital health systems that support a significant proportion of the national priority areas. While most priority areas benefit from these systems, there are still some where digital health solutions are yet to be fully implemented. The existing digital health systems align with public sector priorities and contribute to the advancement of healthcare services. Further efforts are needed to extend the coverage of digital health systems and ensure comprehensive support for all national priority areas. Continuous monitoring and evaluation of these systems are essential to identify gaps and drive improvements.

An example of implemented nationally scaled digital health systems is the key solution provided by the CeZ. This is the P1 e-health System (Electronic Platform for Collection, Analysis, and Sharing of Digital Resources on Medical Events supporting the Medical Information System) and a portfolio of digital products for citizens and medical professionals, which include:

– applications: Internet Patient Account (IKP), myIKP app, gabinet.gov.pl;
– pacjent.gov.pl portal; and
– e-services: e-prescription, e-referral, exchange of Electronic Medical Records, handling of medical events, e-registration for vaccinations, EU COVID Certificate, central e-registration.

Central entity registries collect data on providers, administrators, and public facilities, and support, from the administrative side, the operation of P1 and other IT systems used in healthcare. The essence of these medical registries is that they monitor the demand for healthcare services and the health status of patients, carry out preventive healthcare, implement health programs, and monitor and evaluate the safety, effectiveness, quality, and cost-effectiveness of diagnostic tests or medical procedures. The data collected is not geo-tagged or GIS-mapped.

As part of the CeZ Development Strategy, development work is planned, among other things, for the Registry of Healthcare Providers to implement a technologically newer solution, which is expected to simultaneously improve the system's performance, make it more intuitive, make it more user-friendly, and improve its ergonomics.

There is a universal system, pacjent.gov.pl (patient.gov.pl), which is a centralized database of patients, vaccinations, appointments, prescriptions, and medical activities. The system can be accessed by all Polish citizens and some Ukrainian citizens who have been issued a PESEL personal identification number (Ministry of Health, 2022b). As of November 2022, the system has a recognition rate of 94% and is actively used by 17 million people (e-Health Centre, 2023d), which represents 69% of the adult population of Poland. Data from the system can be accessed by individual patients as well as the specialists providing care.

In addition to building and managing the systems themselves, the CeZ uses the collected data for analytical purposes, supporting management decision-making by institutions responsible for shaping health policy in Poland (e-Health Centre, 2023a, p. 9).

There is a secure birth registry in place maintained within the Civil Status Registry operated by the Ministry of Digital Affairs. The Civil Status Registry identifies civil status records separately for each type of event, including birth records (Ministry of Digital Affairs, 2023). This registry is readily accessible and currently active for health-related purposes. This registry covers over 75% of the relevant population, with data that is available, utilized, and curated. Strategies are being implemented for it to cover 100% of the population.

Additionally, efforts are underway to implement the functionality of generating and storing electronic birth certificates, including annotated stillbirths, in the P1 system. This functionality is scheduled to become fully available for February 1, 2024 (e-Health Centre, 2023c).

A secure death registry is in place. Work is currently in progress to implement electronic death certificates within the e-health system. This development further enhances the accuracy and accessibility of death-related information for efficient healthcare management and reporting purposes.

A secure feedback system exists via the Internet Patient Account (IKP). The patient can fill in an anonymous questionnaire providing feedback on several health procedures such as a consultation with a doctor or a visit to the emergency room.

Thanks to the widespread implementation and ubiquity of digital health tools, huge amounts of data are being generated in Poland. However, the data is still not being put to good use at the level of individual patients and health system employees, or at the level of health management. As part of the implementation of the e-Health Center Development Strategy, an Integrated Analytical Model (ZMA) will be created to embed data in a common environment, ensure a high level of data quality, standardize data, and create consistent definitions for data from different systems, and create an efficient environment to maintain extensive reporting and use by many people. Based on and as part of the ZMA, report dashboards are created and made available to the Ministry of Health and other stakeholders. The ZMA also enables data mining that can then be used for modeling and creating appropriate health policies (e-Health Centre, 2023a; Table 4.8).

Table 4.8 Results summary concerning Services & Applications category in Polish digital health

Indicator No.	Indicator Description	Score	Score Description
19	Nationally scaled digital health systems	4	The majority, but not all national priority areas (50–75% of priority areas) supported by scaled digital health systems.
20	Digital identity management of service providers, administrators, and facilities for digital health, including location data for GIS mapping	3	Health system registries of uniquely identifiable providers, administrators, and public facilities (and private if applicable) are available for use, but incomplete, partially available, used sporadically, and irregularly maintained.
21	Digital identity management of individuals for health	5	A secure registry exists, is available and in active use and includes >75% of the relevant population. The data is available, used, and curated. Strategies are being implemented to include missing data and ensure fully representative datasets are available.
21a	Digital identity management of individuals for health	5	A master patient index exists, is available and in active use and includes >75% of the relevant population. The data is available, used, and curated. Strategies are being implemented to include 100% of the population.

(Continued)

Table 4.8 (Continued)

Indicator No.	Indicator Description	Score	Score Description
21b	Digital identity management of individuals for health	5	A secure birth registry exists, is available and in active use and includes >75% of the relevant population. The data is available, used, and curated. Strategies are being implemented to include 100% of the population.
21c	Digital identity management of individuals for health	5	A secure death registry exists, is available and in active use and includes >75% of the relevant population. The data is available, used, and curated. Strategies are being implemented to include 100% of the population.
22	Secure Patient Feedback Systems	5	A secure feedback system exists, is available in accessible formats and in active use and includes data from >75% of the relevant health services and/or geographic location. It is available to 100% of the population.
23	Population health management contribution of digital health	2	Digital systems used at district/state levels only contribute to public health reporting and decision-making for population health management.

Source: Author's work based on the Digital Health Monitor.

Conclusions

The analyses show that Poland's performance in digital health is generally strong, with an overall performance of 3.45 out of 5. Results from proxy data were higher, at 4.33, but comprehensive comparisons should be treated with caution due to discrepancies and incomplete data.

Poland often matches or surpasses the scores of other developed countries, particularly in Leadership & Governance, Strategy & Investment, Standards & Interoperability, Infrastructure, and Services & Applications. Areas for improvement include Legislation, Policy, & Compliance, and particularly Workforce development. The comparison is presented in Figure 4.1. The list of developed countries used to calculate the average was based on the United Nations HDI data (UNDP, 2022).

Poland boasts a well-established and fully functional governance structure for digital health, overseen by the government with crucial roles assumed by the Ministry of Health and the e-Health Centre (CeZ).

The integration of digital health into Poland's national healthcare strategy is evident through prioritization and inclusion in key strategic documents, which encompass essential aspects, including patient engagement, care coordination, and the advancement of AI and telemedicine tools. Despite

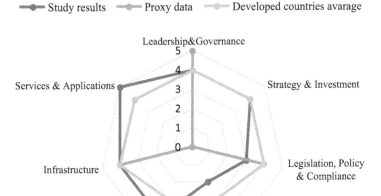

Figure 4.1 Digital health maturity overview for Poland: proxy data, study results
Source: Authors' work based on the Digital Health Monitor.

preparedness for emerging technologies in healthcare, transparency concerns arise from the lack of updates and public reporting on progress.

To systematically address potential benefits and risks, Poland is incorporating digital health into national digital transformation and data governance policies, emphasizing cybersecurity, medical data protection, minimization of disparities in access to digital health services, and human rights impact assessments.

Poland has an approved and costed national digital health plan that sets strategic directions and priorities. Aligned with UHC goals, the plan emphasizes integration, data-driven decision-making, and the establishment of a proficient digital health center. However, there are no metrics to assess the contribution that digital health makes to UHC goals.

While public funding for digital health exists, it is moderately insufficient to fully meet the country's needs. Private sector participation is systematic but falls short, necessitating additional investment and collaboration.

As an EU member state, Poland adheres to the General Data Protection Regulation (GDPR), although implementation and enforcement are inconsistent.

Laws safeguarding individual privacy in digital health data exist, yet implementation and enforcement vary. Protocols for connected medical devices and digital health services are in place but not fully implemented. Cross-border data security and exchange protocols align with EU recommendations but await full implementation.

There is a notable gap in the training given to healthcare professionals on digital health in Poland, with limited coverage in training programs. There are currently no dedicated training programs and career paths for digital health professionals.

Although there is room for improvement in adopting healthcare information standards, Poland's digital health architecture, exemplified by the CeZ architectural repository, aligns with international standards. The Network Readiness Index attests to Poland's substantial network readiness.

The plan for expanding and maintaining digital health infrastructure in Poland is implemented only partially and inconsistently, with 25–50% of necessary infrastructure available. Nationally scaled digital health systems cover priority areas, but efforts are required for wider implementation. Registries for providers and public facilities exist but are incomplete. Digital identity management excels, and a secure feedback system actively contributes to healthcare service improvement.

Poland is actively working on effectively utilizing generated data, with plans for an Integrated Analytical Model.

The Digital Health Profile of Poland presented in this chapter can serve as a foundation for future in-depth research in each specific area and as a valuable resource for policymakers, decision-makers, and health economists.

References

Brewer, L. P. C., Fortuna, K. L., Jones, C., Walker, R., Hayes, S. N., Patten, C. A., & Cooper, L. A. (2020). Back to the future: Achieving health equity through health informatics and digital health. *JMIR MHealth and UHealth, 8*(1). https://doi.org/10.2196/14512Desveaux, L., Soobiah, C., Bhatia, R. S., & Shaw, J. (2019). Identifying and overcoming policy-level barriers to the implementation of digital health innovation: Qualitative study. *Journal of Medical Internet Research, 21*(12). https://doi.org/10.2196/14994

Digital Health Monitor. (2023, June 29). *Methodology.* https://monitor.digitalhealth-monitor.org/methodology

Directive 2011/24/EU of the European Parliament and of the Council of 9 March 2011 on the application of patients' rights in cross-border healthcare (2011). https://eur-lex.europa.eu/legal-content/EN/TXT/PDF/?uri=CELEX:32011L0024&from=EN

e-Health Centre. (2023a). *e-Health Centre Strategy for 2023–2027* [in Polish]. https://cez.gov.pl/sites/default/files/paragraph.attachments.field_attachments/2023-06/strategia_rozwoju_cez_wcag_05.06.pdf

e-Health Centre. (2023b). *e-Health Centre: About us.* https://cez.gov.pl/pl/main-page-en

e-Health Centre. (2023c). *e-Karta Zgonu oraz e-Karta Urodzeń.* Ezdrowie.Gov.Pl.

e-Health Centre. (2023d, April 3). *17 000 000 x IKP.* Pacjent.Gov.Pl. https://pacjent.gov.pl/aktualnosc/17-000-000-x-ikp

European Commission. (2023). *Electronic Cross-border Health Services.* https://health.ec.europa.eu/ehealth-digital-health-and-care/electronic-cross-border-health-services_en

European Parliament. (2023, June 14). *MEPs Ready to Negotiate First-ever Rules for Safe and Transparent AI.* https://www.europarl.europa.eu/news/en/press-room/20230609IPR96212/meps-ready-to-negotiate-first-ever-rules-for-safe-and-transparent-aiFatehi, F., Samadbeik, M., & Kazemi, A. (2020). What is digital health? Review of definitions. *Studies in Health Technology and Informatics, 275,* 67–71. https://doi.org/10.3233/SHTI200696

Gentili, A., Failla, G., Melnyk, A., Puleo, V., Di Tanna, G. L., Ricciardi, W., & Cascini, F. (2022). The cost-effectiveness of digital health interventions: A systematic review of the literature. *Frontiers in Public Health, 10*(2022). https://doi.org/https://doi.org/10.3389/fpubh.2022.787135

Jandoo, T. (2020). WHO guidance for digital health: What it means for researchers. *Digital Health, 6.* https://doi.org/10.1177/2055207619898984Kruse, C. S., Soma, M., Pulluri, D., Nemali, N. T., & Brooks, M. (2017). The effectiveness of telemedicine in the management of chronic heart disease – A systematic review. *JRSM Open, 8*(3), 205427041668174. https://doi.org/10.1177/2054270416681747

Liaw, S. T., Zhou, R., Ansari, S., & Gao, J. (2021). A digital health profile & maturity assessment toolkit: Cocreation and testing in the Pacific Islands. *Journal of the American Medical Informatics Association, 28*(3), 494–503. https://doi.org/10.1093/jamia/ocaa255

Lin, Y. K., Lin, M., & Chen, H. (2019). Do electronic health records affect quality of care? Evidence from the HITECH act. *Information Systems Research, 30*(1), 306–318. https://doi.org/10.1287/isre.2018.0813

Mechael, P., & Edelman, J. K. (2019). *The State of Digital Health 2019.*

Medycyna Prywatna. (2022, October 11). *Strategic Partnership between Lux Med Group and SGH [in Polish].* https://medycynaprywatna.pl/strategiczne-partnerstwo-grupy-lux-med-i-sgh/Ministry of Digital Affairs. (2023, June 2). *Register of Civil Status* [in Polish]. Gov.Pl. https://www.gov.pl/web/cyfryzacja/rejestr-stanu-cywilnegoMinistry of Health. (2021a). *Healthy Future. Strategic Framework for the Development of the Health Care System for 2021–2027, with an Outlook to 2030 [in Polish].* https://www.gov.pl/attachment/4a9bd160-e052-4a52-8fd4-b7c546d556f8

Ministry of Health. (2021b). *National Health Programme 2021–2025 [in Polish].* https://www.gov.pl/web/zdrowie/narodowy-program-zdrowia-2021-2025

Ministry of Health. (2022a). *Program for the Development of eHealth in Poland [in Polish].* https://www.gov.pl/attachment/e491641d-a291-42de-af01-8439600dccc1

Ministry of Health. (2022b, March 17). *IKP dla obywateli Ukrainy.* Pacjent.Gov.Pl. https://pacjent.gov.pl/aktualnosc/ikp-dla-obywateli-ukrainy

Ministry of Health. (2023). *Awarding the Application the Title of 'MZ Certified Application' and Inclusion in the 'Portfolio of Health Applications' (PAZ) through POPI [in Polish].* Portal Obsługi Projektów Inwestycyjnych. https://e-inwestycje.mz.gov.pl/wybranykonkurs/?id=054eb66d-7fc9-ed11-b597-000d3aaaee06

National Reform Programme 2023/2024 (2023). https://commission.europa.eu/system/files/2023-04/Poland_NRP_2023_pl.pdf

Neumann, S. (2015, September 11). *Response to Interrogatory No. 33262 on the Closing Balance of the Health Ministry of Health Operations [in Polish].* Sejm Rzeczypospolitej Polskiej. https://www.sejm.gov.pl/sejm7.nsf/InterpelacjaTresc.xsp?key=75B1759A&view=null

OECD. (2016). *Universal Health Coverage and Health Outcomes.* https://www.oecd. org/health/health-systems/Universal-Health-Coverage-and-Health-Outcomes-OECD-G7-Health-Ministerial-2016.pdf

Order of the Minister of Health dated June 4, 2020 on the e-Health Centre [in Polish] (2020). https://dziennikmz.mz.gov.pl/DUM_MZ/2020/42/akt.pdf

Pokrzycka-Walczak, M. (2023, January 10). *Andrzej Osuch: Digital Solutions Play an Important Role in Making Medical Services More Accessible [in Polish].* SerwisZOZ.Pl. https://serwiszoz.pl/praktycy-radza/andrzej-osuch-rozwiazania-cyfrowe-odgrywaja-wazna-role-w-zwiekszaniu-dostepnosci-uslug-medycznych-7437.html

Policy for the Development of Artificial Intelligence in Poland from 2020. Appendix to the Resolution no. 196 of the Council of Ministers of 28 December 2020 (item 23) (2020). https://www.gov.pl/attachment/928200fa-b1a6-4c0c-b3a8-d1fbf1e1175a

Portulans Institute. (2022). *Network Readiness Index 2022 Poland.* https://networkread-inessindex.org/wp-content/uploads/reports/countries/poland.pdf

Regulation (EU) 2016/679 on the protection of natural persons with regard to the processing of personal data and on the free movement of such data, and repealing Directive 95/46/EC (General Data Protection Regulation), 1 (2016). https://eur-lex.europa.eu/legal-content/EN/TXT/HTML/?uri=CELEX:32016R0679#ntr1-L_2016119EN.01000101-E0001

Regulation of the Minister of Science and Higher Education of July 26, 2019 on the standards of education preparing for the profession of a doctor, dentist, pharmacist, nurse, midwife, laboratory diagnostician, physiotherapist and paramedic (2019). https://isap.sejm.gov.pl/isap.nsf/download.xsp/WDU20190001573/O/D20191573. pdf

Resolution of the Council of Ministers of March 30, 2021 on National Health Programme 2021–2025 [in Polish] (2021). https://isap.sejm.gov.pl/isap.nsf/download. xsp/WDU20210000642/O/D20210642.pdf

Resolution No. 24 of the Council of Ministers of February 21, 2023 on the establishment of a government program called the 'Digital Competence Development Program' [in Polish] (2023). https://isap.sejm.gov.pl/isap.nsf/download.xsp/WMP20230000318/ O/M20230318.pdfRieke, N., Hancox, J., Li, W., Milletarì, F., Roth, H. R., Albarqouni, S., Bakas, S., Galtier, M. N., Landman, B. A., Maier-Hein, K., Ourselin, S., Sheller, M., Summers, R. M., Trask, A., Xu, D., Baust, M., & Cardoso, M. J. (2020). The future of digital health with federated learning. *Npj Digital Medicine, 3*(1). https://doi. org/10.1038/s41746-020-00323-1

Sanocki, A. (2021, May 25). *Three years with GDPR Behind Us [in Polish].* Urząd Ochrony Danych Osobowych. https://archiwum.uodo.gov.pl/pl/138/2059

The Act of 10 May 2018 on the Protection of Personal Data (2018). https://uodo.gov. pl/en/file/754

The Act of 28 April 2011 on the information system in healthcare [in Polish] (2011). https://isap.sejm.gov.pl/isap.nsf/download.xsp/WDU20111130657/U/D20110657Lj. pdf

The Act of 7 April 2022 on medical devices (2022). https://isap.sejm.gov.pl/isap.nsf/ download.xsp/WDU20220000974/T/D20220974L.pdf

UNDP. (2022). *Human Development Report 2021/2022. Uncertain Times, Unsettled Lives: Shaping Our Future in a Transforming World.* https://hdr.undp.org/system/ files/documents/global-report-document/hdr2021-22pdf_1.pdf

WHO. (2023, June 29). *Universal Health Coverage (UHC)*. https://www.who.int/news-room/fact-sheets/detail/universal-health-coverage-(uhc)

Williams, G. A., Fahy, N., Aissat, D., Lenormand, M.-C., Stüwe, L., Zablit-Schmidt, I., Delafuys, S., Le Douarin, Y.-M., & Muscat, N. A. (2022). Covid-19 and the use of digital health tools: Opportunity amid crisis that could transform healthcare delivery. *Eurohealth, 28*(1), 29–34.

Zielonacki, B. (2019, August 26). *NFZ, Medicover and LUX MED are Looking for Start-ups to Collaborate on the Introduction of Digital Solutions* [in Polish]. Termedia. https://www.termedia.pl/wartowiedziec/NFZ-Medicover-i-LUX-MED-szukaja-start-upow-do-wspolpracy-przy-wprowadzaniu-cyfrowych-rozwiazan,35229.html

5 Teleconsultations in Poland

Will the COVID-driven Popularization of Teleconsultations Turn into a Long-Lasting Strategy?

Barbara Więckowska,
Monika Raulinajtys-Grzybek
and Katarzyna Byszek

Introduction

In today's healthcare systems, supply constraints and queues pose significant challenges that impact the timely delivery of patient care. These constraints can lead to long waiting times, delayed diagnoses, and inadequate access to healthcare professionals, ultimately affecting patient outcomes. In an effort to make healthcare services more efficient and accessible, technological solutions have emerged as potential remedies. Remote consultation, also known as telemedicine or telehealth, has garnered considerable attention as a promising solution to address these supply constraints and queues. The primary goal of this chapter is to explore the current role of remote consultations in the Polish healthcare system and its potential to alleviate the challenges posed by supply constraints and queues within healthcare systems.

The concept of remote consultation involves the use of technology to facilitate the delivery of healthcare services remotely, allowing patients to interact with healthcare professionals without the need for physical presence. Using telecommunications tools such as video calls, phone calls, or online messaging platforms, patients can seek medical advice, receive diagnoses, and even obtain treatment recommendations from the comfort of their homes. By leveraging remote consultation, healthcare providers can extend their reach to patients in remote or underserved areas, reduce the burden on physical facilities, and optimize the utilization of healthcare resources.

Given the potential benefits, remote consultation has gained increasing popularity in recent years. It was particularly relevant during the ongoing global pandemic, where social distancing measures and overburdened healthcare systems meant that healthcare had to be provided by alternative means. However, while remote consultation offers promising solutions, its implementation and

DOI: 10.4324/9781032726557-8

effectiveness in mitigating supply constraints and queues within healthcare systems warrant further exploration.

The rapid introduction of remote consultations during the global pandemic era was primarily driven by the urgent need to ensure continuity of care while minimizing the risk of viral transmission. However, this widespread adoption occurred without comprehensive institutional and organizational preparation, as the focus was on immediate implementation rather than long-term planning. As we move forward, it is essential to assess the sustainability and longevity of this trend. The question arises as to which areas of remote consultations will remain prevalent and where patients and healthcare professionals may opt to return to traditional face-to-face consultations.

This research article aims to delve into this question, exploring the factors influencing the preference for remote or in-person consultations and the implications for healthcare systems. By examining the experiences and perspectives of healthcare professionals in Poland, this study seeks to shed light on the future trajectory of remote consultations and guide policy decisions and resource allocation in healthcare delivery.

The State of the Art

Remote consultations have witnessed a significant surge in popularity in recent years. This trend was further accelerated by the COVID-19 pandemic, which necessitated alternative means of providing healthcare (Vidal-Alaball et al. 2020). Studies have shown that patients have embraced remote consultations due to their convenience, accessibility, and ability to overcome geographical barriers. Research by Koonin et al. (2020) revealed a 154% increase in telehealth visits during the early stages of the pandemic in the US, highlighting the rapid adoption and acceptance of remote consultations by both patients and healthcare providers.

Remote consultations were beneficial to healthcare delivery in several ways. A study published in the *Journal of Telemedicine and Telecare* (Cottrell et al., 2018) found that remote consultations significantly improved access to care related to the management of chronic musculoskeletal conditions. The study highlighted the potential of telemedicine to bridge geographical barriers and increase healthcare accessibility for patients who would otherwise face challenges in accessing in-person consultations. Patients can receive timely medical advice, diagnoses, and treatment recommendations without the need for physical travel or face-to-face visits, as shown in the study by Dorsey et al. (2010) and Liddy et al. (2016). Remote consultations also led to reduced waiting times for patients, making provision of healthcare more efficient, as evidenced by studies such as that by Bashshur et al. (2016).

Remote consultations helped to reduce waiting times for patients. By offering virtual appointments and eliminating the need for travel and physical presence, healthcare providers were able to accommodate more patients efficiently, leading to shorter waiting times and improved patient satisfaction (Pinar et al., 2021). Patients appreciate the convenience, reduced travel time and costs, and the ability to access healthcare from their own homes. Research by Wade et al. (2010), Bashshur et al. (2016), and Polisena et al. (2010) demonstrated high levels of patient satisfaction with telemedicine encounters.

Furthermore, numerous studies have shown that remote consultations can achieve comparable clinical outcomes to traditional face-to-face consultations, particularly in areas such as chronic disease management, mental health, and post-operative care. Flodgren et al. (2015) showed that the use of telemedicine in the management of heart failure appears to lead to similar health outcomes as face-to-face or telephone delivery of care; there is evidence that telemedicine can improve the control of blood glucose in those with diabetes.

Remote consultations have shown promising cost-effectiveness in healthcare delivery. Several studies have demonstrated potential cost savings associated with telemedicine. Wade et al. (2010) and Polisena et al. (2009) conducted systematic reviews of economic evaluations and concluded that telemedicine interventions can be cost-effective, particularly in terms of reduced travel expenses for patients and healthcare providers. By minimizing the need for physical infrastructure and streamlining administrative processes, remote consultations can contribute to overall cost savings while maintaining or even improving patient outcomes. Other research however did not produce any substantial evidence that telemedicine is a cost-effective means of delivering healthcare (Whitten et al., 2002). However, it is important to consider specific contexts and conditions under which telemedicine is implemented to fully assess its cost-effectiveness. Factors such as reimbursement policies, technology infrastructure, and patient population characteristics can influence the economic impact.

While remote consultations apply to a wide range of medical conditions, certain factors influence their suitability. The effectiveness of remote consultations may depend on many different factors, including those related to the severity of the condition and the disease trajectory of the participants, and whether it is used for monitoring a chronic condition, or to provide access to diagnostic services (Flodgren et al., 2015). They are most effective for non-emergency situations and routine follow-ups, where physical examination may not be essential. Conditions such as chronic disease management, mental health consultations, dermatology, and minor acute illnesses have been successfully addressed through remote consultations.

However, conditions requiring complex procedures or physical examinations may still necessitate in-person visits, as highlighted by research by Shore et al. (2018). Research indicates that there is still a demand for face-to-face consultations in certain situations. Yee et al. (2022) highlighted that patients and healthcare professionals often preferred in-person consultations for complex or sensitive medical issues that require physical examination or a more personal connection. Those studies emphasize the importance of a balanced approach, integrating remote consultations where appropriate while preserving the value of face-to-face interactions.

Telehealth might also exacerbate existing inequities, because of disparities in broadband and technology access (Barbosa et al., 2021). Technical issues, such as poor internet connectivity or limited digital literacy among patients, as well as technical challenges for staff, can hinder the smooth delivery of telemedicine services (Kruse et al., 2018). Privacy and security concerns related to the exchange of sensitive patient information online also need careful consideration. Additionally, the lack of physical interaction in remote consultations may limit the healthcare provider's ability to perform a thorough examination and can result in misdiagnosis or incomplete assessments (Hjelm, 2005). Studies by Portnoy et al. (2020) and Hollander and Carr (2020) emphasize the importance of mitigating these risks through appropriate safeguards and training.

The popularity and widespread use of remote consultations have prompted the development of regulatory and legal frameworks to ensure safe and effective telemedicine practice. Many countries have established guidelines and policies to govern telehealth services, including requirements for licensure, patient consent, privacy protection, and reimbursement. Research by Gagnon et al. (2016) highlights the importance of well-defined regulations to ensure standardization, quality assurance, and patient safety in remote consultations.

Legal Framework for Remote Consultations in the Polish Healthcare System

The possibility of using information and communication technologies (ICT) in the provision of healthcare services in Poland was introduced in December 2015. This enabled the development of telemedicine, including teleconsultations (Mazurkiewicz & Klich, 2017).

Despite the legal possibility of providing healthcare through teleinformatics or communication systems, there was a practical issue in the public sector regarding the legal basis for settling telemedical services (Sikorski & Florczak, 2019). This was due to the lack of appropriate healthcare services that were publicly funded. Regarding a broad range of teleconsultations, the National Health Fund (NFZ) only contracted telecardiology and telegeriatrics as separate services, involving remote consultations between a primary care physician and a specialist in the respective field. In November 2019, remote consultations were introduced in primary healthcare (Rozporządzenie Ministra Zdrowia z dnia 31 października, 2019). From that time onwards remote consultations could be provided through teleinformatics or communication systems – both by physicians as well as nurses and midwives (Ministerstwo Zdrowia, 2020).

The National Health Fund (NFZ) announced that teleconsultations could be used in specialized ambulatory treatment (AOS) through communications issued in early March 2020 (NFZ, 2020). The third-party payer encouraged the use of this form of healthcare in response to the epidemiological situation associated with the COVID-19 pandemic. Remote visits applied to selected procedures within the scope of specialized healthcare, and they were allowed for patients continuing their care in a specific specialist clinic according to an established treatment plan and clinical condition (Zarządzenie Nr 182/2019/ DSOZ, Regulation of October 31, 2019).

Regarding hospital treatment, teleconsultations were also introduced as a response to the evolving COVID-19 pandemic. However, teleconsultations in this context were relatively limited in scope and were primarily applicable to follow-up visits for stable patients continuing their treatment according to an established therapeutic plan within drug programs and chemotherapy.

Uncertainty regarding the possibility of using teleconsultations arose under Article 9 of the Code of Medical Ethics (CME), which states: "A physician may commence treatment only after a prior examination of the patient. Exceptions are situations where medical advice can only be provided remotely." This wording would suggest that remote consultation is only possible in exceptional situations, as medical law interprets "prior examination" as personal contact between the physician and the patient (Zoń, 2019). Such an interpretation may pose a challenge for physicians who are required to practice their profession in accordance with the principles of professional ethics and, in cases of non-compliance, may face disciplinary proceedings. However, the same set of deontological norms gives physicians the freedom to practice in accordance with their conscience and contemporary medical knowledge (Article 4 of the CME). Therefore, the CME needs to be revised and adapted to the current legal framework for telemedical services.

Another important legal issue regarding the provision of teleconsultations is the matter of the healthcare provider's liability for medical errors. In the absence of specific regulations pertaining to remote consultations, it should be assumed that the same legal principles apply as in the case of in-person care (Telemedyczna Grupa Robocza, 2020). This means that the healthcare provider bears professional, civil (compensatory), and criminal responsibility. The obligation to maintain professional liability insurance also remains in effect.

General practitioners (GP) are financed in the Polish healthcare system on a per capita basis, so in the case of teleconsultations, there is no additional financing for such services. On the contrary, due to the excessive use of teleconsultations leading to an overwhelming influx of patient complaints, the legislature has introduced financial incentives aimed at reducing this form of healthcare services. These incentives were based on three mechanisms: (1) if a family doctor provides no more than 25% of consultations in the form of teleconsultations, they will receive a 5% bonus, (2) if the share of teleconsultations exceeds 75%, the remuneration for the Primary Healthcare Facility (POZ) will be reduced by 10%, (3) if the teleconsultation rate exceeds 90%, the contract with the respective POZ will be terminated without observing the notice termination period.

In the case of specialist ambulatory care, teleconsultation is treated as a basic on-site visit, with the same payment level, and this means that they do not cover the cost of any medical tests. In the case of other services, as there have been no formal changes in legal systems, all types of services on-site or teleconsultations can be declared with no difference in payment level between these forms.

Methods

Mixed-method research was carried out. Hypotheses were formed and initially tested using quantitative data, and then further analyzed during the qualitative part of the study. The interviews provide more long-term conclusions, as the quantitative data shows the trend during the pandemic, and the interviews were performed in Spring 2023.

Data on the provision of healthcare services is analyzed using the statistics for all providers financed by a public third-party payer in Poland. We provide data divided according to the type of services (primary care, ambulatory care, rehabilitation, long-term care, palliative care) and by patients' characteristics (age, sex, place of residence). The time period considered was established as the time from the introduction of financial products (2020/mid-2020) to the time of availability of public information (2021).

The qualitative part of the research was based on findings from in-depth interviews with healthcare providers involved in teleconsultations. The interviews were conducted in 2023 personally by the researcher based on an interview questionnaire. The interviewees included a GP, an ambulatory care specialist, a psychotherapist, and a palliative care specialist. Each of the interlocutors was interviewed individually, and the conversations were digitally recorded. In total, they lasted approximately 30 minutes.

Results

Analysis of data on public healthcare services shows that the COVID-19 pandemic accelerated the development of telemedicine in Poland. A significant impact can be observed in both primary care (GP) and specialized areas such as outpatient specialist care (AOS), psychiatric care, long-term care, and palliative-hospice care. However, the proportion of telemedical services in the overall number of home and outpatient rehabilitation services remained negligible, not exceeding 0.27% in 2021.

Since September 2020, GPs have been required to report teleconsultations using a separate service code enabling them to be identified and analyzed. From September to December 2020, the number of teleconsultations in the GP sector reached 15.6 million, with an average proportion of 28.23% . As the pandemic's intensity diminished, a decrease in the proportion of teleconsultations in the overall number of GP consultations was observed (Figure 5.1). In 2021, this proportion was 24.32%, with a total of 39.57 million teleconsultations. However, the last value includes data for a full 12-month period, whereas the value for 2020 only covers four months. Assuming uniform monthly distribution of services for 2020 (ceteris paribus), approximately 46.8 million such services would have been provided over 12 months, significantly more than in 2021. However, it is important to consider the methodological limitations of this approach, as services provided by a GP are subject to seasonal fluctuations (Figure 5.1).

Findings from the in-depth interview with the physician, who has over eight years of experience in a primary care facility, show that teleconsultations were mostly used during the pandemic, but in 2023 their use tailed off.

The variation in teleconsultation use across age groups confirms the findings of previous systematic reviews. The highest proportion of such services is among individuals aged 19–50 years (Table 5.1). However, the decline in the proportion of teleconsultations in 2021 compared to 2020 was not consistent across age groups (the highest decline was observed among children aged 0–6 years), while in the oldest age group (above 90 years), the proportion of teleconsultations increased by two percentage points.

During the in-depth interview, the primary care physician also stressed that the demand for teleconsultations was driven by a lack of time to travel to the

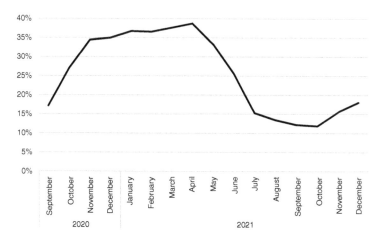

Figure 5.1 Share of teleconsultations in the total number of GP services by month (September 2020–December 2021)

Source: Authors' work based on data from Maps on Health Needs.

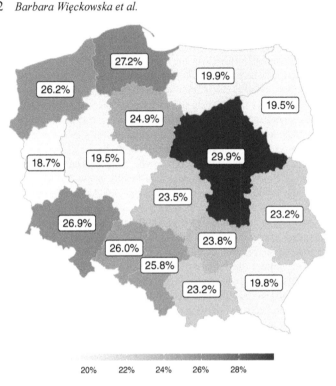

Figure 5.2 Share of teleconsultations in the total number of GP services by voivode-ship (2021)

Source: Authors' work based on data from Maps on Health Needs.

Table 5.1 Share of teleconsultations in the total number of GP services by age groups (2020–2021)

Age Group	2020	2021	Difference
0–6	21.72%	14.15%	−7.57pp
7–18	26.19%	21.99%	−4.20pp
19–30	33.02%	29.09%	−3.93pp
31–40	33.54%	29.81%	−3.73pp
41–50	32.49%	28.65%	−3.84pp
51–60	29.66%	25.93%	−3.73pp
61–70	27.11%	24.25%	−2.86pp
71–80	26.04%	23.54%	−2.50pp
81–90	25.74%	25.09%	−0.65pp
90+	25.61%	27.87%	2.26pp

Source: Authors' work based on Maps on Health Needs.

facility among younger patients and loneliness among the more advanced age groups of patients:

- *Sometimes, patients insist on consultations, especially young people who lack time to travel to the clinic and those who occasionally exaggerate symptoms. In such cases, they are called in for a personal visit.*
- *Many patients, especially older ones, also have a need for contact and conversations with doctors, driven by loneliness due to the loss of a partner, for example. Hence, some of these physical consultations stem from mental needs.*
- The findings from the interview also suggest that there are barriers to maintaining teleconsultations after the pandemic. According to the primary care doctor:
- *[Lack of] Societal change and healthcare reform are key barriers. Teleconsultation actually requires more time, because preparation is needed to inquire about everything that we can immediately determine during an in-person consultation. It takes longer because we have to have longer conversations, better clarify, specify, and ask further questions. Especially with older individuals, we need to dictate and ensure that the patient has heard and understood. Primary care doctors also serve as educators, and health promotion and education are important, but they are hindered or impossible during teleconsultations. It is also difficult to transfer these tasks to nurses because there is resistance from both sides – patients prefer doctors, especially specialists.*
- *During the pandemic, we switched to teleconsultations, but only via telephone. There was no time for other methods. There are no consultations with cameras or video calls, and I wonder how that would work with older individuals who are not familiar with those technologies on a daily basis, so that could be a problem.*

However, teleconsultations in primary care can be beneficial *for older patients with chronic illnesses who have children or other people present during a teleconsultation on a speakerphone. This is an important convenience as it saves travel time and allows them to consult with the doctor, which would also be beneficial for health preventive check-ups.*

In the case of outpatient specialist care (AOS), the average share of teleconsultations in Poland was 14.8% in 2020 and 8.4% in 2021, indicating an almost 43% year-on-year decline (Figure 5.3). Spatial analyses show significantly greater variation between voivodeships compared to primary care consultations, although the voivodeships at each end of the scale remain unchanged. The lowest proportion of teleconsultations was observed in the Lubuskie Voivodeship (4.8%), while the highest was observed in the Mazowieckie Voivodeship (10.4%) (Figure 5.4).

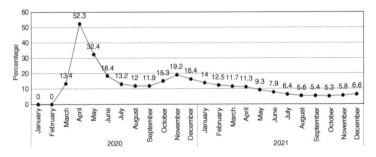

Figure 5.3 Share of teleconsultations in the total number of AOS services by month (2020–2021)

Source: Authors' work based on data from Maps on Health Needs.

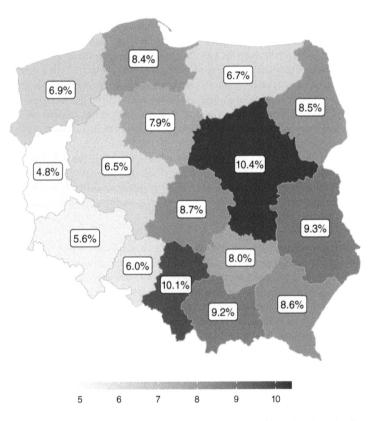

Figure 5.4 Share of teleconsultations in the total number of AOS services by voivodeship (2021)

Source: Authors' work based on data from Maps on Health Needs.

The in-depth interview with the physician with over 30 years of experience in pulmonology, who works in ambulatory care facilities, provided arguments explaining these trends. The epidemiologic situation had the greatest impact on the share of teleconsultations in the total number of consultations in ambulatory care in 2020. Later, as more people were vaccinated, the volume of teleconsultations was reduced:

– *About 70% of consultations during the initial wave of the pandemic were conducted via telemedicine. However, the percentage of patients utilizing teleconsultations gradually decreased by approximately 10% each month, so that by the end of the year, teleconsultations accounted for only around 10–15% of the total. (...)*

The specialist also observed that patient preferences also play an important role in maintaining the level of teleconsultation use, which is not always suitable to their health condition: *Some patients who have become familiar with the option of teleconsultations even demand this type of consultation for unrelated cases, which has its pros and cons. Patients who live at a certain distance may forgo in-person visits due to the effort required for transportation and attempt to seek advice via phone, often in an inaccurate or incomplete manner. They may request, for example, antibiotics over the phone or downplay their symptoms, or demand referrals without physical examinations, or even try to obtain sick leave without an in-person examination. Their knowledge is often based on internet sources and may not be adequate for their actual health condition, leading to a delay in diagnosing potentially serious diseases due to overlooking early symptoms.*

There were several barriers to the wide adoption of teleconsultations in ambulatory care indicated by the pulmonology specialist:

– *Teleconsultations somewhat deviate from the humanistic approach inherent in in-person visits to the doctor. The patient-doctor contact is essential because the patient feels cared for. Establishing such a relationship over the phone is much more challenging than through personal contact. Many older patients complain that they feel lost in computers and codes at present, and they miss the personal contact with the doctor.*
– *During a teleconsultation, we rely on what the patient tells us and their level of observation to detect any symptoms. When we see the patient in person, we can notice things that they may not observe in their daily life, such as changes in skin color or peculiar behaviors, which may not have caught their attention. Therefore, transitioning solely to teleconsultations without the ability to fully utilize the diagnostic capabilities offered by the clinic would be a mistake.*
– *A significant portion of medical personnel are also in an advanced age group and may struggle with the full digitalization that currently exists in healthcare.*

– *[financial barriers] Regarding the financial aspect, the reimbursement for teleconsultations is the same as for regular consultations in the office without any additional physical examination.*

The average proportion of telemedical services in adult psychiatric care in 2021 was 40% (Table 5.2). The majority of these services (over 1.5 million) were observed for medical consultations and individual psychotherapy. In the case of psychiatric care for children and adolescents, the proportion of all telemedical services was much lower – 13% with the highest rate of individual psychotherapy (Table 5.3).

A significant geographical variation in telemedical forms is also observed. The highest share of telemedicine services is observed in the Pomorskie and Śląskie Voivodeships, accounting for approximately 50%. Conversely, the lowest share, 29%, is observed in the Kujawsko-Pomorskie Voivodeship (Figure 5.5).

The findings from the in-depth interview with the psychotherapist with over ten years of experience working with patients in healthcare providers – both out- and inpatient settings that have a contract with the National Health Fund – suggest that several factors influenced patient volume:

– New patient pathways and financing *"During the pandemic, it turned out that some services could indeed be provided remotely. However, in terms of psychiatric or psychotherapeutic services in the public healthcare system, specialists had never had such a solution available before. Previously, it was considered unacceptable in any way. Therefore, the procedure for providing services via this method was devised in such a way that for a new patient, an initial in-person visit was required, especially for evaluation by a psychiatrist. As therapists, we continued to see patients who were already in therapy, and new patients were not [eligible] for therapy during that closed period of the pandemic and lockdown."*

Table 5.2 Structure of services in psychiatric care services for adults (2021)

Type of Health Service	On-site Services	Remote Services	Share
Crisis intervention	17,231	4,449	21%
Remote addiction treatment – teleconsultation		2	100%
Group/family treatment	21,811	2,317	10%
Medical consultation	2,173,390	1,597,982	42%
Psychological consultation	580,979	282,708	33%
Individual psychotherapy	565,162	357,945	39%
Home visits	38,440	332	1%
Total	3,397,013	2,245,735	40%

Source: Authors' work based on Maps on Health Needs.

Table 5.3 Structure of services in psychiatric care services for youth and children (2021)

Type of Health Service	On-site Services	Remote Services	Share
Group/family treatment	236,723	14,753	6%
Medical consultation	698,909	94,588	12%
Psychological consultation	552,038	120,559	18%
Individual psychotherapy	290,558	74,848	20%
Home visits	225,659	1,724	1%
Total	2,003,887	306,472	13%

Source: Authors' work based on Maps on Health Needs.

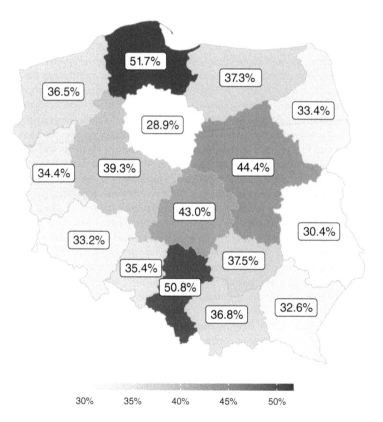

Figure 5.5 Share of teleservices in the total number of psychiatric care services for adults by voivodeship (2021)

Source: Authors' work based on Maps on Health Needs.

– Recommendations on teleconsultations linked to the epidemiological situation: *There were fluctuations, and at times, restrictions were relaxed, resulting in a reduced sense of danger. At the beginning of the pandemic, everything was closed, and contact was very limited. We worked remotely with patients we knew. Then we adopted an approach where we had in-person appointments for initial visits, and subsequent visits were conducted remotely. This approach proved successful. However, later, there was a recommendation to avoid using teleconsultations, and appointments were required to be in person.*

The findings from the interview also helped to understand the needs and nuances of the use of teleconsultations in psychotherapy by different groups of patients: *(...) when it comes to patients, especially those of school-age or preschool-age, or even younger, who sometimes seek assistance from clinics, and lately, much more frequently, remote contact is practically impossible, in my opinion. In the case of young children, establishing relationships and working with them becomes challenging. Additionally, the diagnostic process itself is hindered. It is difficult for me to imagine providing support or therapy for a child in such a remote form. However, with elderly persons, we have noticed that teleconsultations were maintained, and there was even an increase during the pandemic. I think this was due to several factors. One factor was that elderly persons were the group most at risk for various complications from the coronavirus, and illness could have more drastic consequences for them compared to younger individuals or children. Another factor is that older individuals may have other limitations related to mobility or somatic health, and sometimes an online consultation is more comfortable and meets their needs directly.*

Another important insight from the interview was the role of direct engagement with the patient: *We [psychiatric professionals] prioritize direct contact, as it brings much more to the treatment process and provides a more comprehensive form of interaction. However, I do not exclude the possibility that there are many other tele-informatic solutions that could enable equivalent remote contact and may be more widely utilized in the future, now that there is a gateway for teleconsultations. But in the field of psychological or psychiatric care, it will not replace the full range of services.*

The interview with the psychotherapist also was useful in understanding the barriers to maintaining teleconsultations in psychiatric care:

– *Sometimes, it is necessary to carefully consider whether a teleconsultation reinforces someone's fear, such as anxiety about interacting with another person. In such cases, providing services through teleconsultations can be ethically problematic because it does not actually help the person but instead reinforces their fear, leaving them alone with the very problem they sought help for. If we rely solely on remote services, we may exacerbate the patient's disorders. Therefore, the choice of form of consultation should*

not be based solely on the patient's preference but on a comprehensive assessment of their psycho-physical condition.
– There are patients who pose certain challenges, and by agreeing to avoid
  in-person visits, we may reinforce certain symptoms. In such cases, it is
  necessary to have direct contact during the initial stage of therapy and
  make a precise diagnosis. This cannot be done through a computer screen,
  in my opinion.
– Contact through messengers or phone calls always has its limitations because we cannot see each other. We don't know if silence on the other end
  of the line is a natural part of the conversation or if someone has been
  disconnected. There may also be issues with reception, especially when
  additional difficulties with the connection arise, which are not present in
  face-to-face contact.

Despite the barriers listed above, there were also benefits from using teleconsultations, such as convenience and continuity of care:

– It is beneficial for patients to be allowed to have online consultations,
  especially when a patient's health condition prevents them from coming to
  the facility, such as having a fever or facing various systemic obstacles in
  reaching the facility. There is also the possibility of using computer-based
  consultations, where patients can connect with us via a communicator
  with a camera, or on the telephone.
– I think this [teleconsultation] is a huge convenience when it comes to short
  specific cases that concern the continuation of treatment, the issuance of
  prescriptions, or that really concern some trivial cases.

In the case of long-term care (LTC), the proportion of telemedical services
ranged from 2% to 11% with a decreasing trend in individual months of 2021.
However, an analysis of services by type shows significant variation, particularly in the area of medical consultations (Figure 5.6).

Similar conclusions can be drawn when analyzing telemedical services
in palliative-hospice care. The average proportion of telemedicine solutions
within this form of care in 2021 was 19% (Table 5.4). The main contribution
to this indicator came from home visits by nurses, as their proportion in all
open care services in the analyzed scope amounted to over two-thirds. However, for certain services, the proportion of teleconsultations was significantly
higher. For example, among psychological consultations in outpatient care, it
reached 37%.

The in-depth interview with the physician with over 20 years of experience
in palliative care in oncology in publicly funded facilities helped to understand
the trends in use in palliative care facilities: *Teleconsultations appeared in our
practice, like everywhere during the pandemic, but they did not catch on at
all because patients needed to be examined, and they had to be qualified for*

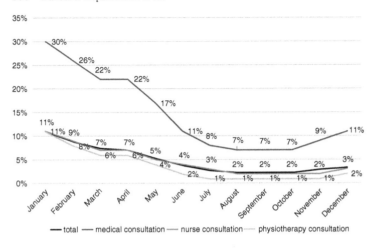

Figure 5.6 Share of teleconsultations in the total number of long-term care services by type and month (2021)

Source: Authors' work based on Maps on Health Needs.

chemotherapy, so exceptions were not considered. In the oncology clinic, teleconsultations were used in cases where prescriptions, test orders, or results of analysis could be sent without the need for direct communication with the patient, which happened occasionally, but they were not generally accepted.

Findings from the interview with the palliative care professional suggest that there are barriers in the wider use of teleservices in palliative care:

– *The first issue is that remote care needs to be evaluated and the price needs to be determined by the National Health Fund because it involves work, such as returning home from a hospital or clinic and sitting in front of a computer, for example, to read all the messages received throughout the day. The second issue is that I would see a solution in providing educational support for caregivers in their own homes, specifically in terms of their ability to connect using a camera. For instance, through a video station where we can at least see each other to some extent – although we can't physically touch the patient, I can see them, and by talking to me, they may derive some benefits like finding comfort. Unfortunately, such knowledge is not widespread among caregivers.*
– *[in palliative medicine], online communication means connecting with both the family and the patient. However, both sides need to have technical readiness, and often there is a problem with that. Both sides simply lack such skills, and we are still learning, as this is relatively new. In general, there were no teleconsultations before the pandemic, and I don't recall any teleconferences or similar things taking place in healthcare facilities.*

Table 5.4 Structure of services in palliative and hospice care (2021)

		Remote Services	On-site Services	Share
Ambulatory care	Consultation	15,020	36,563	29%
	Medical consultation	12,464	25,567	33%
	Nurse visit	1,939	11,209	15%
	Psychologist consultation	1,307	2,230	37%
Home care	Nurse visit	382,448	1,635,770	19%
	Medical consultation	141,943	419,036	25%
	Psychologist consultation	14,288	32,455	31%
	Physiotherapist consultation	10,213	231,691	4%
Ambulatory care	Total	30,730	75,569	29%
Home care	Total	548,892	2,318,952	19%
Total	Total	579,622	2,394,521	19%

Source: Authors' work on Maps on Health Need.

However, according to the palliative care professional, benefits from digitalization and teleconsultations can be observed: *One such selected case where it could be used was electronic communication for sending referrals or prescriptions, and conducting phone conversations to clarify something. It proved effective in situations where telemedicine truly worked, but it is not a universal method and is not suitable for all situations.*

Discussion

The transition to teleconsultation poses challenges due to societal changes, healthcare system reforms, increased time requirements, limitations in education and preventive care, resistance to nurse involvement, and some patients' preference for specialist care over primary care (Carrillo de Albornoz et al., 2022). We have identified several barriers to maintaining and further developing teleconsultations.

The legal framework significantly affects the possibility of using teleconsultations. Introducing teleconsultations only for certain basket cases creates discrepancies in interpretation regarding which areas qualify for reimbursement of such services and which do not. Including telemedicine services in statutory regulations meant that they could be funded in all areas during the COVID-19 pandemic period. However, this should be considered a temporary solution. The absence of provisions in lower-level acts (regulations) means that healthcare providers may be reluctant to invest in technologies and train staff with regard to teleconsultations.

The method of financing teleconsultations also significantly influences their widespread adoption. This is not the case in primary care (POZ), where teleconsultations are considered a statistical service (included in the capitation rate), but there are challenges in using such services in the current reimbursement system for outpatient care. Typically, the first outpatient visit takes place at the provider's premises, and after the physical and subjective examination, as well as the ordering of medical tests, the patient has a follow-up visit. Only during this subsequent visit can the costs of the conducted tests be settled. Healthcare providers use various reimbursement products (ambulatory DRG) that include on-site consultations, making it difficult to use teleconsultations in this context (Co w Zdrowiu, 2020). Teleconsultation is considered a separate financial product, and therefore cannot be easily incorporated. Such a structure of financial products practically limits its usage to cases involving prescription continuation. In such situations, a doctor can conduct an interview remotely, prescribe medication, and settle the teleconsultation accordingly.

According to the Digital Economy and Society Index (DESI) reports Poland is less digitalized than the EU average (DESI). Poland ranks 24th out of 27 countries according to the digital skills benchmark. Only 43% of individuals aged 16 to 74 possess basic digital skills, and 57% have basic digital content creation skills, both below the EU averages. The deployment of Internet infrastructure in Poland also faces challenges, with only 34% of households covered by 5G technology in 2021, ranking 25th in the EU for connectivity. However, there has been progress in increasing the coverage of Fixed Very High-Capacity Networks and Fiber-to-the-Premises technology, particularly in rural areas (European Commission, 2023). The Polish Digital Transformation Strategy for 2025 aims to ensure that all households have internet access with minimum speeds of 100 Mbps, with the possibility of upgrading to gigabit speeds. To achieve this goal, financial and legislative measures are outlined in the National Broadband Plan, addressing barriers to broadband network development. However, the plan does not currently align with the goals of the Commission proposal for the Digital Decade policy program, and an update is planned for 2022. In terms of mobile connectivity, Poland's coverage of 5G technology is currently at 34.2%, below the EU average, mainly due to the absence of a designated radio spectrum for 5G deployment (European Commission, 2023). In the integration of digital technology in business activities, Poland ranks 24th among EU countries. This shows that more effort needs to be made to reach the 2030 Digital Decade target of at least 75% of enterprises taking up cloud services, Big Data, and AI. Finally, Poland ranks 22nd in the EU on Digital public services, and 55% of internet users relied on e-government services (up from 49% in 2021), coming slightly closer to the EU average of 64% (European Commission, 2023). The use of e-government services, including the patient portal, thrived in the wake of the changes in both demand and supply brought about by the COVID-19 pandemic. The patient portal – Internet Patient Account – allows patients, after logging in, to perform most of the essential activities, such as e-prescription consultation, registering for their vaccinations, or specifying a person authorized to access the account.

Findings from one poll of September 2020 suggested that Poles generally have a negative attitude toward telemedicine. Merely 25% of the respondents expressed a preference for telephone or online consultations, while three-quarters of the participants believed that teleconsultations cannot replace in-person visits to the doctor (ARC Rynek i Opinia, 2020). A significant portion, 63%, of Poles state that non-COVID-19 patients received inadequate treatment during the pandemic. Irrespective of the respondents' age, nearly half of them admit to having no faith in telemedicine and consider online or telephone visits to be entirely ineffective (ARC Rynek i Opinia, 2020). Patients need to discuss the health issues they are seeking help for clearly and comprehensibly with their primary care physician to ensure patient safety. Therefore, the National Health Fund conducted a survey on patient satisfaction with teleconsultations. The results from a survey conducted in mid-2020 suggested that 80% of patients were satisfied with teleconsultations, and most respondents were satisfied with receiving complete information about the doctor's recommendations, additional tests that need to be conducted, how to take medication, and where to seek further treatment (NFZ, 2020, *Report on the satisfaction …*). This finding applied to nearly 97% of the respondents. Only about 2% of the surveyed patients reported receiving incomplete information, such as not being informed about the cause of their symptoms, how to take medication, or when to schedule a follow-up consultation. Additionally, only 1.3% of the respondents did not receive satisfactory information regarding their reported health issue (NFZ, 2020, *Report on the satisfaction …*).

Teleconsultations are proposed as a potential solution to a long-standing social problem, geographic disparities in healthcare (Hwang et al., 2017). However, there is little information about the reasons for the differences in the use of teleconsultations across different regions of Poland.

Our research findings help to fill the existing gap. Our analysis provides promising evidence that teleconsultations can improve access to healthcare, specifically by introducing digital education services and redirecting resources from well-equipped regions to underserved areas. This shift is important in addressing the existing healthcare disparities offline. The results highlight the potential of teleconsultations to overcome geographical limitations, i.e., in ensuring transportation to the healthcare facilities and making effective use of available resources. However, alongside these encouraging findings, we also discovered various factors that hinder the flow of teleconsultations. Specifically, social and information barriers arising from demographic and educational differences, as well as limited infrastructure, restrict the seamless movement of teleconsultations within regions and between them.

According to a study conducted in Poland during the pandemic in Lower Silesia, significant differences emerged in terms of time spent on teleconsultation −38% (N=83) report that this form of contact takes less time than a traditional visit, 44% report that it takes more time, and 18% report that it takes the same amount of time (Grata-Borkowska et al., 2021). This is consistent with the findings from the in-depth interviews. According to the interviewees, there is a lot of administrative work that is not included in the reimbursement but is directly linked to the teleconsultations as they may require additional time for documentation and record-keeping. Healthcare providers need to accurately document the consultation details, including patient history, symptoms discussed, diagnoses, prescriptions, and any recommendations. Additionally, physicians need time to prepare for the teleconsultation to make sure that they collect all information that is not obtained just by seeing a patient in person. Our interviewees stressed that in-person consultations allow physicians to conduct a comprehensive physical examination of the patient, which may involve palpation, auscultation, or other hands-on assessments. In teleconsultations, the healthcare provider's ability to perform a thorough physical examination is limited, and they may need to rely more on patient-reported symptoms, which can take additional time and can be exaggerated by patients. Therefore, effective communication is crucial in healthcare interactions. In teleconsultations, there may be challenges in conveying information clearly and interpreting non-verbal cues due to limitations in video or audio quality. Healthcare providers may need to spend extra time ensuring that they understand the patient's concerns, explaining diagnoses or treatment plans, and addressing any misunderstandings.

These challenges are often accompanied by technical difficulties. Teleconsultations rely on technology such as video conferencing platforms, internet connections, and devices. Technical issues, such as poor internet connection, audio or video lag, or software glitches, can disrupt the flow of communication, leading to delays and requiring additional troubleshooting time. Before a teleconsultation, both the healthcare provider and the patient need to ensure they have the necessary technology and setup in place, and as we heard during the interviews – it is not always the case. This may involve support from relatives or tech support in the healthcare facility, downloading and installing software, testing audio and video settings, and familiarizing themselves with the teleconsultation platform. This setup process can add extra time compared to the straightforward process of an in-person consultation.

Teleconsultations are an effective alternative to face-to-face consultations for many patients receiving primary care and mental health services and our research findings suggest benefits such as time-saving for patients who work and would not have time to have consultations if they were required in-person. However, as with any other method of healthcare delivery, there are disadvantages related to teleconsultations, and patients' preferences should not be the only factor when choosing this form of healthcare delivery. This was emphasized in the context of psychiatric care. Many studies suggested that professional perception was likely the greatest barrier to the implementation of telepsychiatry, with clinicians reporting concerns about the therapeutic alliance, data security, and confidentiality (Sharma & Devan, 2023). This was also noted during the interview with the psychotherapist. Another area in which there are additional limitations on the use of teleconsultations is palliative care. One of the main problems in this field of medicine and care is that teleconsultations may not be able to provide the same level of emotional support as face-to-face consultations. Patients with advanced illness may require more emotional support than can be provided through teleconsultations. Both experts who were interviewed stressed that direct contact with the caregiver is the "healing ingredient." However, with technological progress being made at a pace like never before, it cannot be excluded that in the near future there will be technology available that will facilitate assessments equal to hands-on examinations and be a true equivalent of the in-person consultation. Nevertheless, all stakeholders need to be prepared in terms of skills, technology solutions, and procedures along with professional association guidelines to ensure patient safety, address disparities in underserved populations, and ensure the achievement of health outcomes equivalent to in-person care.

Overall, we identified possible mechanisms that contribute to the factors that limit the use of teleconsultations: (1) a financing mechanism that does not differentiate between teleconsultations and in-person consultations, (2) insufficient digital skills of healthcare professionals and patients, and (3) technical and financial constraints faced by patients in underserved areas (like access to equipment with a camera, high-quality internet connection).

Conclusions

Patient safety is the top priority regardless of the field of medicine or form of consultations. Physicians and other healthcare professionals may believe that without physical examination, teleconsultations provide incomplete diagnoses. Teleconsultations rely solely on patient interviews, with no option of conducting a physical examination. This limitation may prevent healthcare professionals from accurately diagnosing certain conditions, potentially leading to suboptimal treatment decisions and a detrimental impact on patient health. The study aimed to explore the factors influencing the provision of remote or in-person consultations to predict the future of remote consultations in Poland.

Our research findings suggest that there is limited accessibility of teleconsultations in some regions. One reason for this could be that in rural areas where there may be only one older doctor, the lack of technological infrastructure and expertise can hinder the implementation of teleconsultations. Medical practices may not have the necessary resources or knowledge to offer teleconsultation services, limiting their adoption.

Teleconsultations pose challenges that can make them more time-consuming than in-person consultations. These include technical difficulties, limited physical examination, communication challenges, setup and preparation time, and documentation requirements. Many older patients may struggle with using computers or digital devices proficiently, which can impede their ability to participate in teleconsultations. Additionally, healthcare professionals, especially older doctors, may face difficulties adapting to the full extent of technological requirements and may require support from IT professionals, which may not always be readily available.

If teleconsultations are not properly implemented, they may result in the loss of the patient-doctor relationship and trust. The personal contact between patients and doctors during in-person visits fosters a sense of care and trust. As they do not have the same level of direct interaction teleconsultations may not be able to produce the same patient-doctor relationship, potentially leading to reduced patient satisfaction and trust in the healthcare system.

Despite the challenges, teleconsultations have shown potential in improving access to healthcare, particularly in addressing geographical disparities. However, factors such as social and information barriers, demographic and educational differences, and limited infrastructure can hinder the widespread adoption of teleconsultations.

While teleconsultations have benefits such as timesaving and accessibility, there are limitations in certain healthcare fields, such as psychiatric care and palliative care, where face-to-face consultations may provide better emotional support. Overcoming these limitations requires advances in technology, skills, and procedures while ensuring patient safety and achieving equivalent health outcomes.

References

ARC Rynek i Opinia. Poles reluctant to telemedicine [Polacy niechętni telemedycynie]. Retrieved July 3, 2023, from http://arc.com.pl/polacy-niechetni-telemedycynie/

Barbosa, W., Zhou, K., Waddell, E., Myers, T., & Dorsey, E. R. (2021). Improving access to care: Telemedicine across medical domains. *Annual Review of Public Health, 42*, 463–481. https://doi.org/10.1146/annurev-publhealth-090519-093711

Bashshur, R. L., Howell, J. D., Krupinski, E. A., Harms, K. M., Bashshur, N., & Doarn, C. R. (2016). The empirical foundations of telemedicine interventions in primary care. *Telemedicine Journal and E-health: The Official Journal of the American Telemedicine Association, 22*(5), 342–375. https://doi.org/10.1089/tmj.2016.0045

Carrillo de Albornoz, S., Sia, K. L., & Harris, A. (2022). The effectiveness of teleconsultations in primary care: Systematic review. *Family Practice, 39*(1), 168–182. https://doi.org/10.1093/fampra/cmab077

Cottrell, M. A., Hill, A. J., O'Leary, S. P., Raymer, M. E., & Russell, T. G. (2018). Patients are willing to use telehealth for the multidisciplinary management of chronic musculoskeletal conditions: A cross-sectional survey. *Journal of Telemedicine and Telecare, 24*(7), 445–452. https://doi.org/10.1177/1357633X17706605

Co W Zdrowiu. (2020, May 14). *Zamieszanie z teleporadą w AOS* [press release]. https://cowzdrowiu.pl/aktualnosci/post/zamieszanie-z-teleporada-w-aos-dla-nfz-placowki-zdezorientowane

Dorsey, E. R., Deuel, L. M., Voss, T. S., Finnigan, K., George, B. P., Eason, S., Miller, D., Reminick, J. I., Appler, A., Polanowicz, J., Viti, L., Smith, S., Joseph, A., & Biglan, K. M. (2010). Increasing access to specialty care: A pilot, randomized controlled trial of telemedicine for Parkinson's disease. *Movement Disorders: Official Journal of the Movement Disorder Society, 25*(11), 1652–1659. https://doi.org/10.1002/mds.23145

European Commission. (2023). *The Digital Economy and Society Index—Countries' Performance in Digitization.* https://digital-strategy.ec.europa.eu/en/policies/countries-digitisation-performance

Flodgren, G., Rachas, A., Farmer, A. J., Inzitari, M., & Shepperd, S. (2015). Interactive telemedicine: Effects on professional practice and healthcare outcomes. *The Cochrane Database of Systematic Reviews, 2015*(9), CD002098. https://doi.org/10.1002/14651858.CD002098.pub2

Gagnon, M. P., Ngangue, P., Payne-Gagnon, J., & Desmartis, M. (2016). m-Health adoption by healthcare professionals: A systematic review. *Journal of the American Medical Informatics Association: JAMIA, 23*(1), 212–220. https://doi.org/10.1093/jamia/ocv052

Grata-Borkowska, U., Drobnik, J., Sobieski, M., Fabich, E., & Bujnowska-Fedak, M. M. (2021, February 20). Use of medical teleconsultations during the COVID-19 pandemic in Poland – Preliminary results. Paper presented at eTELEMED 2021: The Thirteenth International Conference on eHealth, Telemedicine, and Social Medicine.

Hjelm, N. M. (2005). Benefits and drawbacks of telemedicine. *Journal of Telemedicine and Telecare, 11*(2), 60–70. https://doi.org/10.1258/1357633053499886

Hollander, J. E., & Carr, B. G. (2020). Virtually perfect? Telemedicine for Covid-19. *The New England Journal of Medicine, 382*(18), 1679–1681. https://doi.org/10.1056/NEJMp2003539

Hwang, E. H., Guo, X., Tan, Y., & Dang, Y. (2017). Delivering healthcare through teleconsultations: Implication on offline healthcare disparity. Retrieved July 3, 2023, from SSRN: https://ssrn.com/abstract=2988340

Koonin, L. M., Hoots, B., Tsang, C. A., Leroy, Z., Farris, K., Jolly, T., Antall, P., McCabe, B., Zelis, C. B. R., Tong, I., & Harris, A. M. (2020). Trends in the use of telehealth during the emergence of the COVID-19 pandemic – United States, January-March 2020. *MMWR. Morbidity and Mortality Weekly Report, 69*(43), 1595–1599. https://doi.org/10.15585/mmwr.mm6943a3

Kruse, C. S., Karem, P., Shifflett, K., Vegi, L., Ravi, K., & Brooks, M. (2018). Evaluating barriers to adopting telemedicine worldwide: A systematic review. *Journal of Telemedicine and Telecare, 24*(1), 4–12. https://doi.org/10.1177/1357633X16674087

Liddy, C., Drosinis, P., & Keely, E. (2016). Electronic consultation systems: Worldwide prevalence and their impact on patient care-a systematic review. *Family Practice, 33*(3), 274–285. https://doi.org/10.1093/fampra/cmw024

Mazurkiewicz, S., & Klich, A. (2017). *Świadczenie usług medycznych z wykorzystaniem telemedycyny - stan obecny i perspektywy.* In K. Flaga-Gieruszyńska, J. Gołaczyński, & D. Szostek (Eds.), *E-obywatel, E-sprawiedliwość, E-usługi* (pp. 67–82). Wydawnictwo C.H. Beck Warszawa.

Ministerstwo Zdrowia (2020, March 13) *Komunikat Ministra Zdrowia dla podmiotów leczniczych realizujących umowy w rodzaju Leczenie szpitalne programy lekowe oraz Leczenie szpitalne – chemioterapia, a także dla pacjentów objętych tym leczeniem* [press release] https://www.gov.pl/web/zdrowie/komunikat-ministra-zdrowia-dla-podmiotow-leczniczych-realizujacych-umowy

NFZ. (2020). *Raport z badania satysfakcji pacjentów korzystających z teleporad u lekarza podstawowej opieki zdrowotnej w okresie epidemii COVID-19.* https://www.nfz.gov.pl/download/gfx/nfz/pl/defaultaktualnosci/370/7788/1/raport_-_teleporady_u_lekarza_poz.pdf

NFZ (2020, March 11) *Teleporady w ambulatoryjnej opiece specjalistycznej* [press release] https://www.nfz.gov.pl/aktualnosci/aktualnosci-centrali/teleporady-w-ambulatoryjnej-opiece-specjalistycznej,7627.html

Pinar, U., Anract, J., Perrot, O., Tabourin, T., Chartier-Kastler, E., Parra, J., Vaessen, C., de La Taille, A., & Roupret, M. (2021). Preliminary assessment of patient and physician satisfaction with the use of teleconsultation in urology during the COVID-19 pandemic. *World Journal of Urology, 39*(6), 1991–1996. https://doi.org/10.1007/s00345-020-03432-4

Polisena, J., Coyle, D., Coyle, K., & McGill, S. (2009). Home telehealth for chronic disease management: A systematic review and an analysis of economic evaluations. *International Journal of Technology Assessment in Healthcare, 25*(3), 339–349. https://doi.org/10.1017/S0266462309990201

Polisena, J., Tran, K., Cimon, K., Hutton, B., McGill, S., Palmer, K., & Scott, R. E. (2010). Home telemonitoring for congestive heart failure: A systematic review and meta-analysis. *Journal of Telemedicine and Telecare, 16*(2), 68–76. https://doi.org/10.1258/jtt.2009.090406

Portnoy, J., Waller, M., & Elliott, T. (2020). Telemedicine in the era of COVID-19. *The Journal of Allergy and Clinical Immunology: In Practice, 8*(5), 1489–1491. https://doi.org/10.1016/j.jaip.2020.03.008

Regulation of October 31, 2019 *Rozporządzenie Ministra Zdrowia z dnia 31 października 2019 r. zmieniające rozporządzenie w sprawie świadczeń gwarantowanych z zakresu podstawowej opieki zdrowotnej.* Dz.U. 2019 poz. 2120.

Sharma, G., & Devan, K. (2023). The effectiveness of telepsychiatry: Thematic review. *BJPsych Bulletin, 47*(2), 82–89. https://doi.org/10.1192/bjb.2021.115

Shore, J. H., Yellowlees, P., Caudill, R., Johnston, B., Turvey, C., Mishkind, M., Krupinski, E., Myers, K., Shore, P., Kaftarian, E., & Hilty, D. (2018). Best practices in videoconferencing-based telemental health, April 2018. *Telemedicine Journal and E-health: The Official Journal of the American Telemedicine Association, 24*(11), 827–832.

Sikorski, S., & Florczak, M. (2019). Telemedycyna w polskim prawie administracyjnym. In I. Lipowicz, G. Szpor, & M. Świerczyński (Eds.), *Telemedycyna i e-zdrowie. Prawo i informatyka* (pp. 40–65). Wolters Kluwer.

Telemedyczna Grupa Robocza. (2020). *Podstawowe Zasady Udzielania Świadczeń Telemedycznych.* Warszawa.

Vidal-Aballí, J., Acosta-Roja, R., Pastor Hernández, N., Sanchez Luque, U., Morrison, D., Narejos Pérez, S., Perez-Llano, J., Salvador Vèrges, A., & López Seguí, F. (2020). Telemedicine in the face of the COVID-19 pandemic. *Atencion Primaria, 52*(6), 418–422. https://doi.org/10.1016/j.aprim.2020.04.003

Wade, V. A., Karnon, J., Elshaug, A. G., & Hiller, J. E. (2010). A systematic review of economic analyses of telehealth services using real time video communication. *BMC Health Services Research, 10*, 233. https://doi.org/10.1186/1472-6963-10-233

Whitten, P. S., Mair, F. S., Haycox, A., May, C. R., Williams, T. L., & Hellmich, S. (2002). Systematic review of cost effectiveness studies of telemedicine interventions. *BMJ, 324*(7351), 1434–1437. https://doi.org/10.1136/bmj.324.7351.1434

Yee, V., Bajaj, S. S., & Stanford, F. C. (2022). Paradox of telemedicine: Building or neglecting trust and equity. *The Lancet. Digital Health, 4*(7), e480–e481. https://doi.org/10.1016/S2589-7500(22)00100-5

Zarządzenie [Ordinance of December 31, 2019] Prezesa Narodowego Funduszu Zdrowia z dnia 31 grudnia 2019 r. w sprawie określenia warunków zawierania i realizacji umów o udzielanie świadczeń opieki zdrowotnej w rodzaju ambulatoryjna opieka specjalistyczna Nr 182/2019/DSOZ.

Zoń, K. M. (2019). *Stosowanie art. 9 Kodeksu Etyki Lekarskiej w świetle orzecznictwa sądów lekarskich.* In I. Lipowicz, G. Szpor, & M. Świerczyński (Eds.), *Telemedycyna i e-zdrowie. Prawo i informatyka* (pp. 141–163). Wolters Kluwer.

Part 3

Digitalization in Medical Research Practice

6 Adaptation of Time Series Analysis to Central Statistical Monitoring of Clinical Trials

A Pilot Study

Maciej Fronc

Introduction

Clinical trials are an extremely time- and cost-consuming undertaking, and they exploit organizations' resources at different levels of their activity. Clinical trials absorb 58.6% of the research and development expenditures for new drug development (Buonansegna et al., 2014). The number of registered studies rises in supralinear fashion each year (U.S. National Library of Medicine, n.d.), but all of them are at risk of failure in reaching the next phase or final approval. In the case of medicines tested on humans, the probability of failure is 90% in each of these phases (Buonansegna et al., 2014). Hence, potential failure entails a heavy financial loss for the organization responsible for the clinical trial. Moreover, clinical trial costs are rising at a fast rate, whereas the number of approvals has decreased by one-third.

A key role of clinical trials is to provide evidence for the evaluation of new medicines. That is why most of the funds are spent on ensuring that data collected are of adequate quality and they are free from errors (Buyse et al., 2020). Otherwise, the image of the investigated medication may be distorted, which will jeopardize the decision-making process regarding final approval of the new drug. This kind of evidence is provided by monitoring clinical trials, which is a key element of the drug development process. Its basic function is to assure data quality and protocol compliance with respect for patient safety and well-being as a priority. Most companies implement the monitoring strategy based on on-site visits which rely heavily on source data verification (SDV) and source data review (SDR). SDV compares recorded data with the source documentation, and SDR investigates the quality of the source documentation. Although on-site monitoring is implemented routinely, this approach is not as efficient as expected. Fully implemented SDV and/or SDR (100% SDV/SDR) usually reveal only a few errors of significance for the study outcome. What is more, on-site visits with 100% SDV/SDR generate huge costs due to travel and workload

DOI: 10.4324/9781032726557-10

(Stansbury et al., 2022; Venet et al., 2012), which is estimated at 60% of the total clinical trial budget (Buyse et al., 2020).

In response to the aforementioned issue, regulatory agencies and other pharmaceutical-industry-related organizations recommend the risk-based approach, which focuses on 'thing that really matter' (Buyse et al., 2020). This idea was conceptualized to the quality management strategy called *risk-based quality management* (RBQM), which concentrates on risk-bearing activities at a different level of the study (EMA, 2013). A part of this strategy is risk-based monitoring (RBM), where clinical trials are monitored in a manner appropriate to the identified risk. RBM is recognized as an effective and efficient approach to clinical trial monitoring (Oba, 2016). This approach enriches the current practice with centralized monitoring (CM), defined as a remote evaluation of aggregated clinical data conducted using data analytics and visualization to identify any kind of discrepancies and data patterns suggesting a direction of further investigation in terms of risk mitigation. CM is conducted at the point of convergence of several roles – e.g., monitors, data management personnel, or statisticians. The implementation of CM reduces the frequency of on-site visits, produces results that are no worse or even better, and provides additional capabilities compared to monitoring conducted fully on-site (Agrafiotis et al., 2018; FDA, 2013). The daily routine of central monitors strongly relies on Business Intelligence tools that decompose the study conduct into many sub-processes to be visualized on a dashboard for further tracking. RBM combines both CM and on-site monitoring in a different proportion as solutions complementary to each other.

Central statistical monitoring (CSM) is a more specific kind of CM which comes down to providing statistical indicators of quality based on data collected and stored in different repositories associated with a certain study. CSM relies on a data quality assessment across the entire study in order to provide maximum data consistency (Buyse et al., 2020). Venet et al. (2012) formulated three principles of statistical monitoring:

1   Relying on clinical data which are highly structured as a consequence of the same protocol followed by all centers involved in the study, and the same case report form (CRF).
2   The multivariate structure of clinical data and time dependency of variables makes statistical assessment powerful. Univariate statistical analysis is insufficient in terms of discrepancies and patterns (caused by fabrication, falsification of data or just errors) and detection, whereas multivariate statistical analysis is more sensitive to human intervention in the original data.
3   Every clinical variable carries an information load needed to evaluate data quality, not only those associated with predefined quality indicators. These variables require a large number of tests whose results are analyzed in terms of outlier identification.

An opportunity to interfere with clinical data can lead to fraudulent activity, which is a noticeable problem in clinical trials. However, CSM deals with detection of this kind of activity successfully (Oba, 2016). This is another premise to adopt statistical methodology in CM. Fraud detection refers to the second aforementioned principle, as clinical data are hard to produce due to limited comprehension of randomness by humans. As Sakamoto and Buyse (2016) state, CSM is a general investigative tool for identifying problems; however this methodology still needs to be developed by adopting new solutions through cross-fertilization of disciplines (Fronc & Jakubczyk, 2022).

As clinical data are a sequence of values collected over the period of study conduct and intervals between patient visits are not constant, clinical trials can be considered an unevenly spaced time series. Clinical time series are short, as a single study is conducted within a certain phase lasting a few years. As Rousseeuw et al. (2019) stated, unusual patterns such as outliers, level shifts, and structural changes are observable analyzing time series. They propose a method of time series monitoring in order to fraud detection. This method compares the forecast with actual data in terms of discrepancies between them. Any significant differences raise concerns about the reliability of collected data. In turn, Thomakos et al. (2022) addressed short time series in the context of forecasting with limited information. Time series analysis (TSA) is usually used for long-term forecasting based on data from a longer period in the past. However, the nature of data generated nowadays requires a different approach that assumes they are created in shorter periods and the time perspective of the forecast is closer to the present. Butler-Laporte et al. (2020) applied TSA to modeling prescribing habits influenced by the study conduct. Their research is an example of backward analysis in terms of data pattern detection.

The aim of this research was to investigate usability of TSA for CSM. This method was applied to clinical data in order to extract hidden information about the study conduct as a basis for further decision-making. The information provided by the TSA outcome could be an indicator of misconduct in the study.

Methods and Data

All operations on data were implemented in the R package version 4.1.1.

Data

This research was performed on real data[1] from a clinical trial conducted by GSK plc (formerly known as GlaxoSmithKline plc), a British biopharmaceutical company. This study is a randomized phase one trial on oncological medication. The analysis focused only on laboratory variables related to the concentration of molecules present in blood measured for all 112 patients

Table 6.1 Laboratory variables involved in the analysis

Variable Name (molecule measured in blood)	Short Variable Name	Unit
Albumin	ALB	g/L
Calcium corrected for albumin	CACRALB	mmol/L
Hemoglobin	HGB	g/L
Lactate dehydrogenase	LDH	IU/L
Lymphocytes	LYM	10^9/L
Neutrophils	NEUT	10^9/L

Note: IU – international units.

enrolled in the study. Six of them were involved in the research as they were identified by the company's experts as key in this therapeutic area (Table 6.1).

Data Pre-processing

Data used within this analysis were collated in accordance with the study data tabulation model (SDTM) which is a standard structure for clinical trial data-sets and non-clinical ones as well. This framework makes it possible to organize clinical trial information as required by regulatory agencies (CDISC, n.d.; Mabe, 2011). Examples of requirements of the agencies are stated in the Food and Drug Administration's (FDA) guideline regarding electronic submissions in electronic format. The purpose of study data standards is to provide un-ambiguous information exchange between information systems (FDA, 2021). The SDTM can be explained in a more illustrative way where a typical tabulation is structured as follows: an observation per site, per patient, per visit, per item, per another item, etc.

Within a single item, there could be more than one variable collated, which means that any numeric results to be analyzed are nested in a single column. Then they should be split into separate columns using merging conditions or at least grouping by categories. In this case, the data were merged by subject identifiers and visit dates. However, TSA imposed certain requirements resulting in further data pre-processing. TSA requires equal periods between timepoints, which is difficult to ensure in the case of clinical data reported with regard to the day. As medical appointments usually take place more than once a month, the results were averaged over the months separately for each patient. If the monthly inter-vals were still not equal, missing datapoints were interpolated against the nearest values. The performed data transformation was necessary to make TSA feasible.

Correlation Analysis

Correlation between all of the selected variables was examined by comput-ing the Pearson correlation coefficient. Two out of six of the least correlated variables were chosen and included in the TSA in order not to duplicate the same information load by these two items.

Time Series Analysis

Clinical Time Series Diagnostics

The first step of the TSA involves the application of autocorrelation function (ACF) and partial autocorrelation function (PACF) in order to diagnose initially time series in terms of data pattern detections. Clinical data are an example of short time series, which determines a lack of enough periods for graphical decomposition. However, both functions give premises to conclude properties of time series.

The crucial one is stationarity to be confirmed by an augmented Dickey-Fuller (ADF) test. This test was implemented using the `adf.test()` function. Its default settings assume no trend and no constant according to the equation derivate of the first-order autoregressive process

$$\Delta y_t = \delta y_{t-1} + \varepsilon_t \tag{6.1}$$

where $\Delta y_t = y_t - y_{t-1}$, $\delta = \alpha - 1$, and ε_t is white noise. For $|\alpha| < 1$ the process is stationary; in turn, for $\alpha = 1$ it is a first-order integrated process (Gruszczyński et al., 2009). A drawback of that assumption is that stationarity and trend-stationarity are considered one category. In consequence, the function de-trends the process automatically, and the test does not show directly whether the trend is present within the process.

Therefore, researchers recommend to use Equation (2) with the extended deterministic part

$$\Delta y_t = \beta_0 + \beta_1 t + \delta y_{t-1} + \varepsilon_t \tag{6.2}$$

where β_0, β_1 are constants, and t is time (Gruszczyński et al., 2009). These two additional elements can be specified in the `adfTest()` function. However, in terms of trend detection, only the β_0 component should be included, otherwise the function would detrend the process. This functionality was used for determining whether the trend exists.

The next step is completion of the clinical time series diagnostics using characteristics of ETS and ARIMA models. Terms of models are specified by default. All of these terms are chosen to provide the best possible results. These elements are informative in terms of processes observed within clinical data over time. The ETS model provides information on error, trend, and seasonality of the time series, and whether they are additive, multiplicative, or just non-present. In turn, the ARIMA model indicates the order of integration, and a number of model components resulting from autoregressive (AR) and moving average (MA) processes.

Clinical Time Series Forecasting

The data were split into two subsets – training and test subsets. The last six records were separated from the original dataset to create the test set. The rest of the data points were included in the training set. Then, laboratory values were forecast for the next six months and compared with the test data. Forecasting was performed using three models – SES, ETS, and ARIMA. All these models were compared in terms of their accuracy. Models with the best accuracy were plotted again, this time including confidence intervals at the level of 80% and 95%. Test data points were added to these graphs in order to identify outliers which are meaningful in terms of the centralized monitoring practice.

Results

Correlation Analysis and Variable Selection

The correlation analysis verified dependencies between selected six variables. Most of them are low or moderately correlated with each other. These relationships were depicted on the heatmap supplemented by the dendrogram identifying variable clusters (Figure 6.1). The color palette was selected to identify correlated (dark grey color means full correlation) and non-correlated variables (white color means no correlation).

CACRALB and LYM were chosen for the next step of the analysis as the two variables that were most dissimilar.

Clinical Time Series Diagnostics and Forecasting

This step of the analysis was applied on variables CACRALB and LYM covering all patients. However, only two of the most interesting (and diverse) cases were included in further considerations, i.e., patient 2 for CACRALB and patient 192 for LYM.

CACRALB, subject 2

Results for CACRALB, subject 2 were displayed on the simple plot and additional ones presenting ACF and PACF in order to conduct an initial investigation of characteristics of the time series (Figure 6.2).

The process of CACRALB, subject 2 seems to be non-random as there is one significant lag, although most of them are close to zero on the ACF plot. However, it is hard to say whether the process is stationary, as the

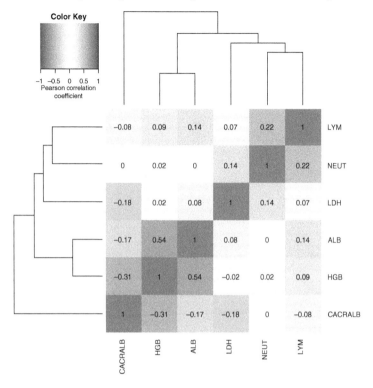

Figure 6.1 Correlation heatmap for selected variables

ACF declines to zero rapidly at lag 2 but increases afterwards. In turn, the ACF seems to fluctuate periodically, which suggests that the seasonal patterns occur, but vaguely. It also means there is no trend. If the trend had existed, the function would have tapered off gradually as a result. In this case, drops are rapid and non-monotonic. Both functions are significant at lag 1, but they do not tail off clearly, which is not an adequate premise to apply a first-order autoregressive model.

Table 6.2 summarizes the results of the ADF test performed with different commands for lag 1. The `adf.test()` function proved stationarity of the process but without details as to the kind. The stationarity was confirmed by the `adfTest()` function, which means no trend exists in that case. The time series seems to be first-order integrated, and no further iterations for other lags are necessary.

In Tables 6.3 and 6.4, ETS and ARIMA models were characterized in terms of their components. In this case, the ETS model defines only error as additive. Other model terms – trend and seasonality – are not present, which

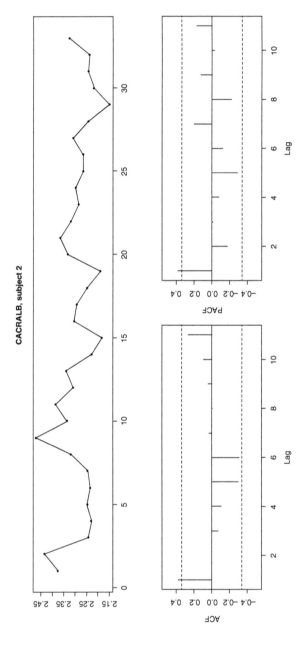

Figure 6.2 Variability over time supplemented with ACF and PACF plots for CACRALB, subject 2

Table 6.2 ADF test results for CACRALB, subject 2

Function	Dickey-Fuller Statistic	p-value	Process
adf.test()	−3.91	0.025	Stationary
adfTest()	−4.04	<0.01	Stationary (no trend)

Table 6.3 ETS model summary for CACRALB, subject 2

Component	Status or Type
Error	Additive
Trend	Non-present
Seasonality	Non-present

Table 6.4 ARIMA model summary for CACRALB, subject 2

Component	Coefficient	p-value
MA1	0.361	0.028
Mean	2.299	<0.01

Table 6.5 Forecast accuracy for CACRALB, subject 2

Model	ME	MAE	RMSE	MAPE	MASE
SES	−0.062	0.070	0.080	3.184%	1.168
ETS	−0.062	0.070	0.080	3.184%	1.168
ARIMA	−0.063	0.072	0.081	3.249%	1.193

is consistent with previous assumptions. In such a case, the ARIMA model has only one MA, which dispels doubts related to the interpretation of ACF and PACF plots. There is also the mean as a constant, which is due to CACRALB fluctuation around a certain level. Both components are statistically significant. However, unlike the ADF test results, the order of integration is zero.

Table 6.5, summarizes the short-term forecast outcome achieved using accuracy measures for all applied models. Accuracy of the models only slightly varies, therefore it is difficult to identify the best model unequivocally. Nevertheless, the SES and ETS models are more accurate than ARIMA. The ME, MAE, and RMSE are close to zero. MAPEs are around 3%, which means the forecast is highly accurate. However, MASE is greater than one, which makes the models worse compared to simple ones.

As Figure 6.3 shows, the ARIMA model varies over time, whereas other models are almost constant. Forecasted curves for SES and ETS models even

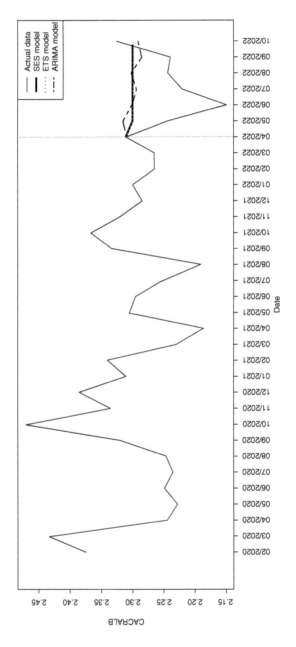

Figure 6.3 Forecast comparison for CACRALB, subject 2

out, and they overlap to a large extent. Although the ARIMA model has the best results, none of the modeled curves converge with the test data.

The ETS forecast was chosen as an example to be plotted with confidence intervals and test data points. Figure 6.4 shows one point exceeding both confidence intervals to be considered as an outlier. The rest of the data points are included in the 80% confidence interval.

LYM, subject 192

The results for LYM, subject 192 were displayed on the simple plot and additional ones presenting ACF and PACF in order to conduct an initial investigation of characteristics of the time series (Figure 6.5).

The trend for the process observed for LYM, subject 192 is quite clear. The ACF is significant for the first five lags; where at least one significant lag suggests a non-random pattern. What is more, the function tails off gradually, which is characteristic for non-stationary time series. The statistical significance of subsequent lags for the ACF tapers off slowly, which clearly demonstrates a trend in this process. The function fluctuates vaguely, indicating seasonality. Both functions tail off, and they have at least one significant lag, and this means the ARMA model can be applicable in this case.

Table 6.6 summarizes the results of the ADF test performed with different commands for lag 1. The `adf.test()` function proved stationarity of the process but without details as to the kind. The stationarity was confirmed by `adfTest()` function, which means that no trend exists in that case. The time series seems to be first-order integrated.

In Tables 6.7 and 6.8, the ETS and ARIMA models were characterized in terms of their components. In this case, the ETS model defines only error and trend terms. Both are additive. The presence of the trend is consistent with previous assumptions. In such a case, the ARIMA model has three AR components and no MA ones. There is also a drift, which is a direct consequence of the trend. All AR terms are statistically significant; in turn, the drift is undoubtedly significant at the level of 0.01. The ARIMA model is consistent with the conclusion provided by the ADF test on the integration order of 1.

Table 6.9 summarizes the short-term forecast outcome using accuracy measures for all applied models. In this case, the ETS model is the most accurate. MEs, MAEs, and RMSEs are greater than zero, but still small enough. None of the MAPEs exceed 10%, which proves adequate accuracy of these models. What is more, MASEs are lower than one, which proves that the models are more accurate than the simple ones.

Figure 6.6 presents forecasts for all three models. The best performance was yielded by the SES model. The model follows the trend but tends to fluctuate as well. From the first forecast timepoint, the ETS model clearly follows the trend of the process as a straight line. In turn, the ARIMA fluctuates the most, which causes the irregular shape of the modeled curve.

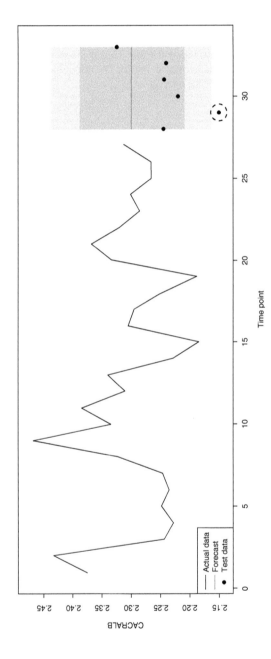

Figure 6.4 Outlier detection for CACRALB, subject 2

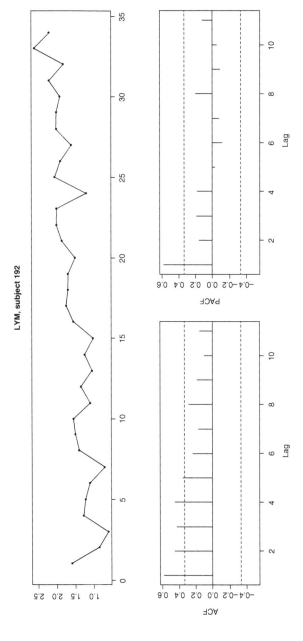

Figure 6.5 Variability over time supplemented with ACF and PACF plots for LYM, subject 192

Table 6.6 ADF test results for LYM, subject 192

Function	Dickey-Fuller Statistic	p-value	Process
adf.test()	−5.23	<0.01	Stationary
adfTest()	−1.44	0.522	Non-stationary

Table 6.7 ETS model summary for LYM, subject 192

Component	Status or Type
Error	Additive
Trend	Additive
Seasonality	Not present

Table 6.8 ARIMA model summary for LYM, subject 192

Component	Coefficient	p-value
AR1	−0.817	<0.01
AR2	−0.708	<0.01
AR3	−0.476	<0.01
Drift	0.036	0.047

Table 6.9 Forecast summary for LYM, subject 192

Model	ME	MAE	RMSE	MAPE	MASE
SES	0.305	0.309	0.402	13.397%	0.974
ETS	0.112	0.205	0.263	9.156%	0.645
ARIMA	0.117	0.217	0.286	9.606%	0.683

The ETS forecast was chosen as an example to be plotted with confidence intervals and test data points. Figure 6.7 shows one point exceeding only the 80% confidence interval, but it still remains in the 95% confidence interval. The rest of the data points are included in the 80% confidence interval.

Discussion

TSA definitely provides hidden information load behind clinical data. As a technique which models phenomena in a time manner, TSA turned out to be applicable in clinical trials.

This research introduced TSA into CSM of clinical trials in two senses. First, as a tool for clinical time series diagnostics which decomposes previous

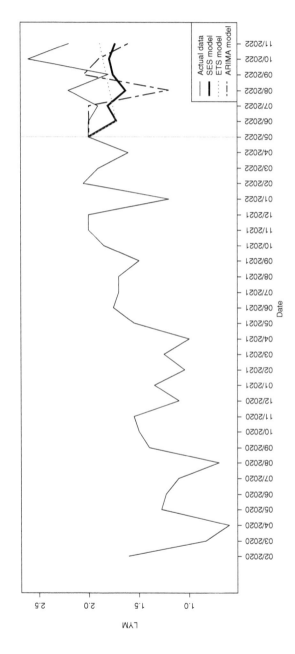

Figure 6.6 Forecast comparison for LYM, subject 192

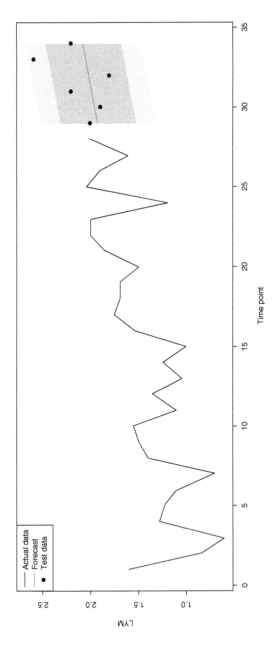

Figure 6.7 Outlier detection for LYM, subject 192

study conduct and facilitates data pattern identification, and second, as a tool forecasting clinical results in the near future. Predicted values might be a reference point for data quality assessment of newly collected results. Additionally, the confidence interval of the forecast points out outliers that could be recognized as 'hot spots' for further on-site investigation. The backward TSA identified trial irregularities at the patient level; in turn, the forward TSA did so at the single observation level.

The context of clinical trials tells us how to interpret the TSA outcome and identify disturbing signals from irrelevant observations. For example, the trend observed in clinical data is undesirable unless it is a natural consequence of the investigated medication. Many laboratory variables fluctuate strongly and their trajectory should resemble a random walk or even white noise. The trend suggests that something atypical has happened. This is a premise for seeking an explanation for this kind of observations by ordering further remote or on-site investigations. The situation is similar with regard to seasonality, which is also an unexpected occurrence.

Every phase of a clinical trial lasts up to a few years. CSM is usually recommended after one year or more until the study reaches an expected study population size. Therefore, it forces the implementation of TSA based on short time series, which is a basic limitation of the method as the information load behind data can be insufficient.

This issue might be solved by using multivariate TSA. As clinical trials are embedded in a high dimensional space, correlated variables could complete the image of the modeled process. Another suggestion for further research is to perform TSA on other clinical variables. It could be performed on data from different studies, but in the same therapeutic area in order to compare trials and seek general rules in this area.

TSA analysis is a promising technique with potential for application in CSM. It helps to investigate the trial with respect to future values and those already collected. The backward analysis provides diagnostics of the clinical time series. In turn, the forward analysis supports the identification of outlying values as a kind of 'traffic light' system. The technique definitely needs to be further developed, being applied to other datasets in order to successfully adopt TSA in daily CSM practice.

Acknowledgement

I would like to thank GSK plc for sharing data for the purpose of this study and their overall support in the implementation of my research project.

Note

1 The human biological samples were sourced ethically and used for research in accord with the terms of the informed consents under an IRB/EC approved protocol.

References

Agrafiotis, D. K., Lobanov, V. S., Farnum, M. A., Yang, E., Ciervo, J., Walega, M., Baumgart, A., & Mackey, A. J. (2018). Risk-based monitoring of clinical trials: An integrative approach. *Clinical Therapeutics, 40*(7), 1204–1212. https://doi.org/10.1016/j.clinthera.2018.04.020

Buonansegna, E., Salomo, S., Maier, A. M., & Li-Ying, J. (2014). Pharmaceutical new product development: Why do clinical trials fail? *R and D Management, 44*(2), 189–202. https://doi.org/10.1111/radm.12053

Butler-Laporte, G., Cheng, M. P., Thirion, D. J. G., de L'Étoile-Morel, S., Frenette, C., Paquette, K., Lawandi, A., McDonald, E. G., & Lee, T. C. (2020). Clinical trials increase off-study drug use: A segmented time-series analysis. *Open Forum Infectious Diseases, 7*(11), 1–5. https://doi.org/10.1093/ofid/ofaa449

Buyse, M., Trotta, L., Saad, E. D., & Sakamoto, J. (2020). Central statistical monitoring of investigator-led clinical trials in oncology. *International Journal of Clinical Oncology, 25*(7), 1207–1214. https://doi.org/10.1007/s10147-020-01726-6

CDISC. (n.d.). *SDTM*. Retrieved June 1, 2023, from https://www.cdisc.org/standards/foundational/sdtm

European Medicines Agency (EMA). (2013). *Reflection Paper on Risk-based Quality Management in Clinical Trials*. https://www.ema.europa.eu/en/documents/scientific-guideline/reflection-paper-risk-based-quality-management-clinical-trials_en.pdf

Food and Drug Administration (FDA). (2013). *Guidance for Industry Oversight of Clinical Investigations — A Risk-based Approach to Monitoring Guidance for Industry Oversight of Clinical Investigations — A Risk-based Approach to Monitoring*. https://www.fda.gov/media/116754/download

Food and Drug Administration (FDA). (2021). *Providing Regulatory Submissions in Electronic Format — Standardized Study Data*. https://www.fda.gov/media/82716/download

Fronc, M., & Jakubczyk, M. (2022). From business to clinical trials: A systematic review of the literature on fraud detection methods to be used in central statistical monitoring. *Przegląd Statystyczny, 69*(3), 1–31. https://doi.org/10.5604/01.3001.0016.1165

Gruszczyński, M., Kuszewski, T., & Podgórska, M. (2009). *Ekonometria i badania operacyjne*. Warszawa: Wydawnictwo Naukowe PWN.

Mabe, B. (2011). SDTM implementation guide – Clear as mud: Strategies for developing consistent companystandards. *CDISC and Industry Standards*, 1–5. https://www.lexjansen.com/phuse/2011/cd/CD02.pdf

Oba, K. (2016). Statistical challenges for central monitoring in clinical trials: A review. *International Journal of Clinical Oncology, 21*(1), 28–37. https://doi.org/10.1007/s10147-015-0914-4

Rousseeuw, P., Perrotta, D., Riani, M., & Hubert, M. (2019). Robust monitoring of time series with application to fraud detection. *Econometrics and Statistics, 9*, 108–121. https://doi.org/10.1016/j.ecosta.2018.05.001

Sakamoto, J., & Buyse, M. (2016). Fraud in clinical trials: Complex problem, simple solutions? *International Journal of Clinical Oncology, 21*(1), 13–14. https://doi.org/10.1007/s10147-015-0922-4

Stansbury, N., Barnes, B., Adams, A., Berlien, R., Branco, D., Brown, D., Butler, P., Garson, L., Jendrasek, D., Manasco, G., Ramirez, N., Sanjuan, N., & Worman, G. (2022). Risk - based monitoring in clinical trials: Increased adoption throughout

2020. *Therapeutic Innovation & Regulatory Science, 56*(3), 415–422. https://doi.org/10.1007/s43441-022-00387-z

Thomakos, D., Wood, G., Ioakimidis, M., & Papagiannakis, G. (2022). ShoTS forecasting: Short time series forecasting for management research. *British Journal of Management*, 1–16. https://doi.org/10.1111/1467-8551.12624

U.S. National Library of Medicine. (n.d.). *Trends, charts, and maps*. Retrieved June 23, 2023, from https://classic.clinicaltrials.gov/ct2/resources/trends

Venet, D., Doffagne, E., Burzykowski, T., Beckers, F., Tellier, Y., Genevois-Marlin, E., Becker, U., Bee, V., Wilson, V., Legrand, C., & Buyse, M. (2012). A statistical approach to central monitoring of data quality in clinical trials. *Clinical Trials, 9*(6), 705–713. https://doi.org/10.1177/1740774512447898

7 Generalized Diffusion Model to Understand and Predict Viral Spread

Paulo H. Acioli

Introduction

Along the history of the world, there were several infection pandemics that had catastrophic consequences. As early as 430 BC an outbreak of typhoid fever was recorded in Greece that is known as the plague of Athens which killed a quarter of the Athenian troops and a quarter of its population (Littman, 2009). Other early history-known pandemics of note are the Antonine Plague (165–180 AD), which were possibly attributed to measles or smallpox that are estimated to have killed 5 million people (Sabbatani, 2009); the Plague of Cyprian (251–266 AD) which is considered to be a second outbreak of what may have been the same disease as the Antonine Plague; the Plague of Justinian (541–549 AD) which is considered to be the first recorded outbreak of bubonic plague that started in Egypt and reached Constantinople, and at its peak, it killed as many as 10,000 people a day resulting the elimination of a quarter to half the known human population at the time (Keller, 2019). Nearly 800 years (1331–1353) after the Plague of Justinian the bubonic plague returned on what is known as the Black Death. The plague returned a few times in England and the population was reduced by 50% by 1370. The last major outbreak of the plague in the second wave was known as the Great Plague of London and is estimated that it killed approximately 20% of its population. The Plague returned in 1855 starting in China and moving to India with a death toll of about 10 million people. The first appearance of the plague in the US was in San Francisco, between 1900 and 1904. In the early 1900s, the Spanish flu infected about half a billion people with a death toll between 20 and 100 million. The Spanish flu, like most influenza outbreaks has the largest death toll in the very young and very old portion of the population. COVID-19 was the most recent event characterized as a pandemic, it started in 2019 in the Hubei province in China, and it started to spread throughout the world in 2020. It is interesting to note that some of the measures taken such as the use of masks and lock downs received the same resistance as the Spanish flu. There were other significant events such as the Ebola virus in 2014 and the SARS outbreak of 2002 that put the world in the state of alert and led to the creation of response protocols and/or agencies to deal with possible widespread health

DOI: 10.4324/9781032726557-11

events. Widespread health hazards and/or pandemic events have also been the subject of many science fiction books and movies (Brooks, 2006; Crichton, 1969; Defoe, 1772, 2003; Flynn, 1987, 2006; Herbert, 1982; Keyes, 2014; King, 1978; Matheson, 1954; Sigler, 2008; Stewart, 1942; Willis, 1992). These works seem to forecast many of the difficulties that were observed during the COVID-19 pandemic as well as some of the possible measures that were taken to contain it. It is also reasonable to expect that they can be the origin of new conspiracy theories and/or reinforce old ones, thus making it more difficult to respond to these threats (Andrews, 2021).

During the 2014 Ebola outbreak, the US put together a document to respond to high-consequence health threats (National Security Council, 2020). In a recent article (Dangerfield et al., 2023), the authors discuss how mathematical modeling was used to inform three different initiatives to respond to health emergencies in the UK, namely the Virtual Forum for Knowledge Exchange in Mathematical Sciences (V-KEMS), Infectious Dynamics of Pandemic (IDP) research program and Rapid Assistance in Modelling the Pandemic (RAMP). These initiatives are focused on statistical modeling and patterns in the data to make short-term predictions and inform on measures to slow down the risks of a widespread epidemic. Similar statistical analyses are proposed by Yang et al. (2023) where they use different techniques to correct predictions using daily-confirmed cases and death occurrences. In this work, we are interested in physical models to the spread of infectious diseases. A good example is the agent-based model proposed by Pais et al. (2023) in which they considered, geographic characteristics, mobility, age as well as safety measures. This was a very complete model that was able to reproduce the COVID-19 data for Parana City (Entre Ríos, Argentina). In the present work, we further explore a very simple physical model based on the diffusion of particles that was initially proposed to be used in a classroom setting to explain the differences of COVID-19 case rates in the cities of Chicago and New York (Acioli, 2020). It was remarkable that a model based on independent moving people that diffuse over an area according to a Brownian motion was able to qualitatively and quantitatively explain the similarities and differences of the growth rate of cases in the two cities. Here we explore how would the spread of the virus be different if one considers that the mobility might be different in different areas of a town, if travel between cities is allowed, as well as the effect of social distancing.

Methods

The original method (Acioli, 2020) was based on the simple diffusion equation in 2 dimensions (2D)

$$\frac{\partial f(x,y,t)}{\partial t} = D\left[\frac{\partial^2 f(x,y,t)}{\partial x^2} + \frac{\partial^2 f(x,y,t)}{\partial y^2}\right]. \tag{7.1}$$

This equation describes a Brownian motion of a single particle characterized by a diffusion constant D, which we will interpret as the population mobility. The normalized solution to Eq. 7.1 is given by

$$f(x,y,t) = \frac{f_0}{\sqrt{4\pi Dt}} e^{-\frac{x^2+y^2}{4Dt}} . \tag{7.2}$$

This is a Gaussian distribution with zero mean and variance $\sqrt{2Dt}$ and can be readily simulated and generalized to N-independent particles. The original algorithm (Acioli, 2020) is described below. The ingredients in the simulation are the population density ρ, the number of inhabitants (particles in the simulation cell) N_{pop}, the diffusion constant D, the number of simulation steps N_{step}, the time step dt, the incubation period (t_{inc}), the transmission radius (r_{transm}), and the probability of transmission from an infected to a healthy individual (prob). All these variables are set at the beginning of the simulation. Below are the steps in the program:

1 Input N_{pop}, ρ, N_{step}, D, dt, t_{inc}, prob, r_{transm}.
2 Calculate the size of the square cell as $L = \sqrt{N_{pop}/\rho}$.
3 Initialize the population.
4 Choose a fraction of the initial population to be infected, and set timer for the sickness (t_{sick}).
5 Loop over N_{step}.
6 Move all individuals according to the Gaussian distribution (Eq. 7.2).
7 Compute the distance between each healthy and infected individual. If the distance is less than r_{transm}, the healthy individual becomes sick with probability prob.
8 Subtract the sickness timer by dt.
9 If $t_{sick} \leq 0$ the sick individual gets cured.

Since these are statistical simulations, we run it multiple times (typically 20) and average the results.

Results

The tests performed in our prior work (Acioli, 2020) are shown below. Using a 100-people simulation cell and the same diffusion constant ($D = 100$ m²/day) and population densities of Chicago and New York City (0.0047 people/m² and 0.0120 people/m²), we simulate the spread of the virus for a period of 90 days. We show the results of these simulations in Figures 1.1 and 1.2. One can see that the rate of cases in NYC is faster than the number of cases in the city of Chicago, which is an indication that the infection rate is proportional to the population density. This result agrees with the data that shows that the initial growth rates follow an exponential trend with exponents 0.462/day and 0.368/day for NYC and Chicago, respectively. The reason why the number of cases levels off very quickly in the simulations is the small population size and the fact that we assumed short-term immunity for those that have been infected and cured.

The assumption that the diffusion constant is the same in both cities seemed reasonable, however, given that the lower the density the larger the area available to move it is also reasonable to think that the diffusion constant is inversely proportional to the population density. We tested this hypothesis by running multiple simulations with different diffusion constants and compared with the data for Chicago and NYC as presented in our previous work (Acioli, 2020). First, we repeated the simulations with a population of 1,000 individuals and 20 simulation blocks and the same parameters as those shown in Figure 7.1. The results are presented in Figure 7.2. In the prior work, the best data was assuming a transmission rate of 1 m. In the present work, we are using a value of 2 m in accordance with the safety guidelines from the United

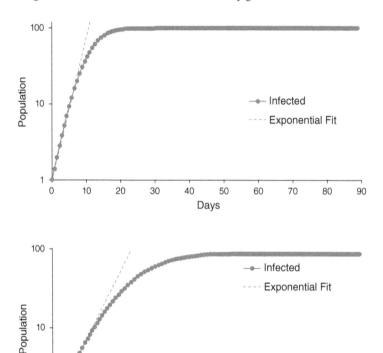

Figure 7.1 The number of infected individuals (full line) in a logarithmic scale and the exponential fit for the initial ten days of the simulation (dashed line) averaged over 50–90-day simulations of the spread of a virus in a population of 100 individuals in a square cell with the population density of the city of (a) NYC (0.0120 people/m²) (b) Chicago (0.0047 people/m²). $D = 100$ m²/day, prob = 0.2, $dt = 0.01$ day, $r_{transm} = 1$ m.

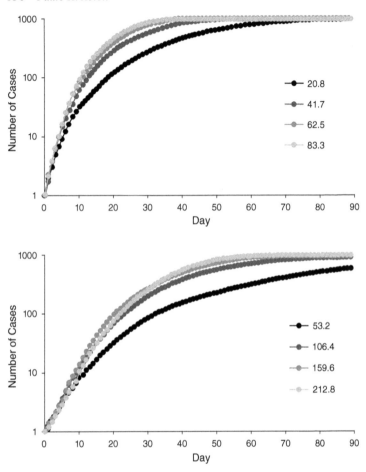

Figure 7.2 The number of infected individuals in a logarithmic scale as a function of the diffusion constant averaged over 20 90-day simulations of the spread of a virus in a population of 1,000 individuals in a square cell with the population density of the city of (a) NYC ($\rho = 0.012$ people/m^2) (b) Chicago ($\rho = 0.0047$ people/m^2). $D = 100$ m^2/day, prob = 0.1, dt = 0.01 day, $r_{transm} = 2$ m.

States Centers for Disease Control and Prevention (CDC). Using the 1,000 individual populations, we obtained exponential growth rates of 0.607 and 0.373, for NYC and Chicago respectively. The growth rate for Chicago is in very good agreement with the real data, while the simulated rate for NYC is 31% larger than the data. This is another indication that the growth rate might be inversely proportional to the diffusion constant.

One can see from Figure 7.2 that the growth rate is proportional to the diffusion constant. To better assess this assertion, we did an exponential fit for the initial growth, since the small size of the population will lead to quick leveling off of the number of cases, we performed an exponential fit for the first 10 days. We present these results in Table 7.1. The rates obtained from the available data for these cities are also presented. Inspection of Table 7.1 shows that the best agreement for both cities is obtained for the diffusion constants of 41.7 and 106.4 m²/day, for the cities of NYC and Chicago, respectively. This corresponds to a $D = 1/(2\rho)$ dependence of the diffusion constant with the population density.

One limitation of the model is that the diffusion process is slow and localized and therefore the spread will go outward from the first case leaving a trail of recovered cases as seen in Figure 7.3. Another limitation is the location of the first sick individual, whether it starts in the center or near one of the corners of the simulation cell, as they will have different numbers of potential neighbors that can come in contact. To more accurately simulate the spread process, we considered travel within each city, by allowing once a day a random traveler per 1,000 people to move randomly over the simulation cell. This process should account for both limitations mentioned above. In Table 7.2 we present the results of the exponential fit as a function of the diffusion constant when considering travel within the city limits. Table 7.2 indicates that the addition of a single random in city traveler does not substantially impact the growth rates.

We considered cities with densities corresponding to New York City and Chicago. The rates obtained from the available data for these cities are also presented.

The next test of the influence of the diffusion constant in the virus spread is to consider a single town (unit cell) that has different diffusion constants. We divided the simulation cell into two equal area cells and different diffusion constants according to Figure 7.4. The first case we considered was an initial uniform density of 0.0047 people/m², corresponding to the city of Chicago,

Table 7.1 Exponential growth rate as a function of diffusion constant for obtained from the first ten days of simulation of 1,000 individuals in cities with densities corresponding to New York City and Chicago

NYC ($\rho = 0.012$ people/m²)			Chicago ($\rho = 0.0047$ people/m²)		
D (m²/day)	Rate	R²	D (m²/day)	Rate	R²
Data	0.462	0.988	Data	0.368	0.969
20.8	0.404	0.965	53.2	0.282	0.993
41.7	0.500	0.944	106.4	0.386	0.980
62.5	0.570	0.904	159.6	0.400	0.995
83.3	0.666	0.666	212.8	0.426	0.994

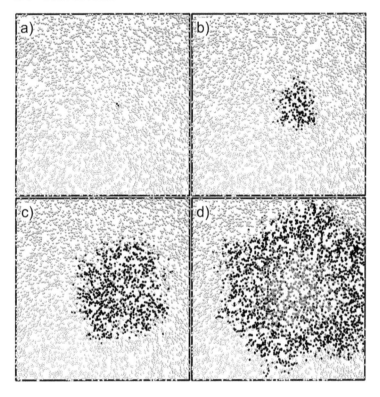

Figure 7.3 Snapshots of a single simulation of 10,000 people arranged in a simulation cell with the density of the city of Chicago. The color-coded spheres correspond to healthy (grey), infected (black), and recovered (light grey) individuals

Table 7.2 Exponential growth rate as a function of diffusion constant for obtained from the first 10 days of simulation of 1,000 individuals with one random traveler per day in each city

NYC ($\rho = 0.012$ people/m^2)			Chicago ($\rho = 0.0047$ people/m^2)		
D (m^2/day)	Rate	R^2	D (m^2/day)	Rate	R^2
Data	0.462	0.988	Data	0.368	0.969
20.8	0.404	0.972	53.2	0.281	0.991
41.7	0.501	0.933	106.4	0.371	0.984
62.5	0.538	0.925	159.6	0.425	0.988
83.3	0.570	0.904	212.8	0.483	0.986

and diffusion constants of 106.4 and 41.7 m^2/day that we found to best yield the observed growth rates for Chicago and NYC, respectively. On the first set of 20 simulations, we placed the first sick person on the high diffusion constant side, and in the next set we placed the first sick person on the low

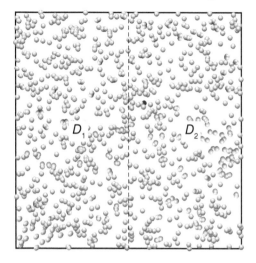

Figure 7.4 Example of a two-diffusion constant simulation cell with 1,000 individuals. The left side of the cell has a diffusion constant D_1 and the right has a diffusion constant D_2. The initial population is uniformly distributed over the whole simulation cell

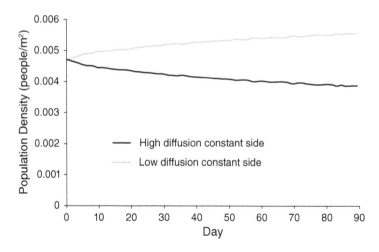

Figure 7.5 Population density as a function of time for a two-diffusion constant simulation cell with initial population density of 0.0047 people/m². The black line represents the high diffusion constant side ($D_1 = 106.4$ m²/day). The grey line represents the low diffusion constant side ($D_2 = 41.7$ m²/day)

diffusion constant side of the simulation cell. In Figure 7.5, we plot the population density on each side of the simulation cell as a function of time. One notes that the population density decreases in the high diffusion constant side and increases in the low diffusion constant side. This reinforces our argument that the population density is inversely proportional to the diffusion constant. To verify this conjecture, we ran a simulation where the initial population density is the 0.00835 people/m², this would allow the low-density region to reach the population density of Chicago and the high-density region to reach the population density of NYC. To allow the system to reach equilibrium, we ran the simulation for 180 days. The results for the population density are presented in Figure 7.6 and although the system did not reach equilibrium the densities after 180 days are 0.0057 and 0.0110 people/m², which are in reasonable agreement with the values of 0.0047 and 0.0120 people/m² corresponding to Chicago and NYC, respectively. We repeated the same simulations for a period of 360 days and the final densities in the two regions were 0.00497 and 0.0117 people/m². This confirms our previous conclusion that the diffusion constant follows the $D = 1 / (2\rho)$ dependence.

In Figure 7.7, we compare the results obtained of the growth rates of the two-diffusion constant simulation cells with the single density simulations using the densities and diffusion constants of the city of Chicago and NYC. The first case in the two-diffusion constant was placed on the high diffusion constant side. It is interesting to note that although as we saw in Figures 7.4 and 7.5 there is a clear change in density in each region, the number of cases for the two-diffusion constant (Town 3) followed very closely the growth rate of the low-diffusion constant high-density town (Town 2).

Our next results are referent to two separate towns with the population densities of Chicago (Town 1) and NYC (Town 2) that can interact by exchanging one random traveler from each city traveling to the other. Our hope

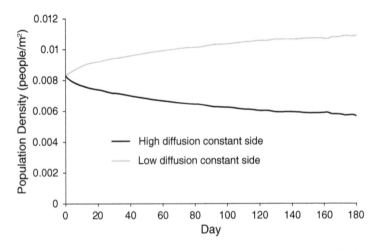

Figure 7.6 Population density as a function of time for a two-diffusion constant simulation cell with initial population density of 0.00835 people/m². The black line represents the high diffusion constant side (D_1 = 106.4 m²/day). The grey line represents the low diffusion constant side (D_2 = 41.7 m²/day)

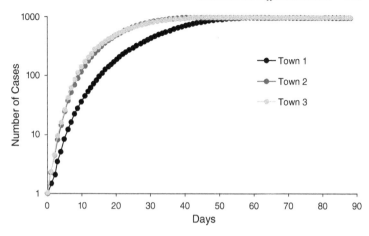

Figure 7.7 Comparison of the number of cases of two towns (Towns 1 and 2) with fixed diffusion constants with a two-diffusion constant simulation cell with initial population density. The black line represents Town 1 ($D_1 = 106.4$ m²/day). The dark grey line represents Town 2 ($D_2 = 41.7$ m²/day). The light grey line represents Town 3 ($\rho_3 = 0.00835$ people/m², $D_1 = 106.4$ m²/day, $D_2 = 41.7$ m²/day)

is to show how an epidemic can be caused by a sick person being one of these random travelers. The total population in each town was 1,000, therefore the rate of traveling was 1 traveler per 1,000 people per day. In the first set of simulations, the first case of the disease was chosen from Town 1. In Figure 7.8, we present the number of cases as a function of time for this case. It is clear that if travel is not restricted the epidemic will eventually spread to Town 2. It is interesting to note that on average the first case has a gap of about three weeks, however in some individual simulations the first case happened on day one of the first case of Town 1, in such cases at the end of 90 days the whole population of Town 2 was eventually contaminated. Another interesting observation was that the initial growth rate in both towns was, on average, similar to what we observed in the isolated town simulations we presented above. Another peculiarity is that the average number of cases in Town 2 seems to level off at a smaller value than in the individual cases. The main reason is that in many of the individual simulations, the random travelers were either healthy or no longer transmitting the disease, and therefore a full epidemic was not observed.

In Figure 7.9, we considered the same two towns; however, the first case of the disease took place in Town 2. As in Figure 7.8, the first case in Town 1 happened about 15 days after the first case in Town 2. In this case, the growth rate for each town follows the same trends as in the simulations of the isolated individual cities, which is proportional to the population density. Once again, the average of cases in the town that did not have an infected individual on day one levels off at a lower value than in the individual cases.

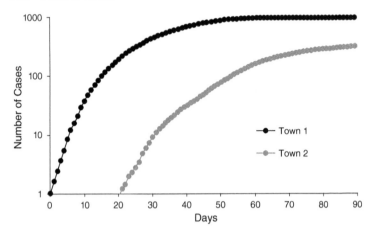

Figure 7.8 Number of cases (in logarithmic scale) as a function of time for a simulation of two interacting 1,000 people towns with the population densities of Chicago (Town 1) and NYS (Town 2). The first contaminated individual was in Town 1

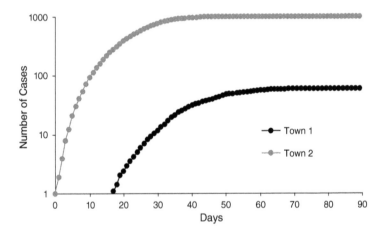

Figure 7.9 Number of cases (in logarithmic scale) as a function of time for a simulation of two interacting 1,000 people towns with the population densities of Chicago (Town 1) and NYS (Town 2). The first contaminated individual was in Town 2

This is attributed to the fact that in some individual simulations, there was no epidemic on Town 1, and in other cases the whole population got infected. In both cases that we considered interacting cities, it is very important to either restrict travel or to closely monitor the travelers to avoid the contamination spreading to other cities.

Discussion

In this chapter, we presented an extension to a simple diffusion model (Acioli, 2020) to study the spread of infectious diseases. The original model was based on individuals moving around the simulation cell in a Brownian motion with a set diffusion constant, and a healthy individual could be infected if it came in contact with a sick individual. The ingredients for this model were the diffusion constant, population density, probability of infection, transmission radius, incubation, and sickness periods. We have originally concluded that the initial growth rate of the number of cases was proportional to the population density and had assumed that the mobility, represented by the diffusion constant, to be the same. A more in-depth study has shown that a quantitative agreement was reached with different diffusion constants for different population densities, suggesting an inverse relationship. Fitting an exponential for the first days of infection allowed us to conclude that the dependence of the diffusion constant with the density followed $D = 1 / 2\rho$, which seems reasonable as there will be less available area to roam around the denser population. These conclusions were drawn from a uniformly distributed population. Our first extension beyond the original model was to consider a cell with regions of different mobility. In this study, we considered half of the region with one diffusion constant, and the other half with a different one (Figure 7.4). To help with the comparison with the results with a single diffusion constant, we used the same population densities and diffusion constants characteristic of the cities of Chicago and New York City. Starting from a uniform density, we observed that the population migrated from the high-diffusion constant to the low-diffusion constant side of the simulation cell, further indicating that the population density is inversely proportional to the diffusion constants. To test this hypothesis we considered an overall initial density that was the average of the cities of Chicago and NYC and using the diffusion constants that led to the best quantitative agreement we indeed showed that given enough time the system will reach equilibrium at the population densities of the individual towns, further confirming our initial finding of the $D = 1 / 2\rho$ relationship between population density and diffusion constant. In this mixed density town the growth rate was very similar to the ones observed in the high-density town. In future studies, we will consider different size areas of different diffusion constants and determine how that will affect the growth rate in the individual regions and for the overall population.

Another possible limitation of the original model is the limited range of motion of each individual. This fact leads to only propagating the disease to people near infected individuals, leading to an outward wave of the disease (Figure 7.3). To overcome this limitation, we allowed some random individuals to randomly travel to any point of the simulation cell. Although that led to the disease spreading all over the cell in a more realistic pattern, the fit to the first 10 days of the disease was hardly affected (Tables 7.1 and 7.2), and the remaining simulations in this study only considered individuals moving on a Brownian like motion within each city.

The next generalization was to consider the effect of travel in spreading diseases to different cities. To simulate this effect, we considered two individual towns (simulation cells) of different density and diffusion constants. To compare with the prior simulations we once again considered the parameters for the cities of Chicago and New York. We placed one sick individual in one of the two towns on day one and allowed one random individual to travel to the other city once a day. Since we considered 1,000 simulation cells, the rate of travel was one traveler per 1,000 inhabitants per day. We averaged the results over 20 different simulations and arrived at the following conclusions: there is a lag of two to three weeks for the first case in the city that started with all healthy individuals. In this case, the first individual started in the low-density town, and the lag was three weeks; when the first case started in the high-density town, the lag was two weeks. This can be explained by the fact that the growth rate is larger at the high-density town. The lag is due to the course of the disease itself, that in this model was a seven-day incubation period, and seven days until the individual recovered. Another observation was that the average of cases in the town that was originally disease free leveled off at values smaller than those in the isolated town simulations. This was due to the fact that in only a fraction of the simulations the epidemic was transmitted to the other town. The ratio of the maximum value obtained in this simulation and the level in which a sick person was placed on day one of the isolated town simulation gives you the probability that the infection due to travel. In the case that we considered 1,000 people towns with the population density of Chicago and NYC, the probability of infection in NYC when the first case was in Chicago was 30%, while the probability of an epidemic in Chicago when the first case happened in NYC was 10%. Nevertheless, with a single random traveler a day per 1,000 people, the model showed that an epidemic would spread to different towns. This makes it clear that travel restrictions and/or travel monitoring are important interventions in case of highly contagious diseases. Very recently Aristov et al. (2023) have done a statistical simulation that does consider some of the elements discussed in this paper, such as travel within regions and travel between different regions. Although this model is statistical in nature, the dependence on population density and mobility is built in the model. The biggest difference is that they treat the high mobility of the disease carriers explicitly.

Our last modification to the original model was to include social distancing by a repulsive force between individuals. To simulate partial compliance this force was attributed to a percentage of the population. We considered a force that was dependent on the square of the distance, after a few tests we obtained the desired effect with $F_{ij} = 2 / r_{ij}^2$, where F_{ij} represents the force between individuals i and j, and r_{ij} represents the distance between them. To isolate the effects of social distancing, we applied social distancing to isolated towns and studied the effects of 25%, 50%, and 75% compliance. Because the addition of the force severely slows down the code, we did the study in a 100-inhabitant town. We studied the effects in towns with low-population density (Chicago), and high-populations density (NYC). The results are presented in Figure 7.10.

One can see that the reduction in the number of cases is felt in both towns, and the larger the compliance level the fewer cases were observed. It is clear that the model supports the common-sense idea of social distancing as a means of avoiding the spread of epidemics.

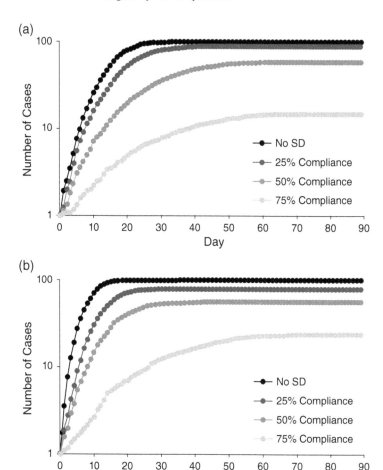

Figure 7.10 Comparison of the number of cases (in logarithmic scale) as a function of time for a simulation of 100 population towns for different social distance levels of compliance. The lines represent different compliance levels: No compliance (black), 25% compliance (dark grey), 50% compliance (grey), and 75% compliance (light grey). The top panel represents a tow with the population density of Chicago. The bottom panel represents a town with the population density of NYC

In summary, we have shown that one can improve on the simple model of using diffusion as a means of spreading viruses adding more realistic elements as well as interventions to contain it spread. In future work, we will consider including isolation as well as the effects of other interventions such as masks and vaccination.

Conclusions and Highlights

In this chapter, we present a physical model of virus spread through a population using a diffusion of subjects on a cell. This is an extension of a simple diffusion model (Acioli, 2020) that was meant as a pedagogical tool for computational physics courses. The original model has shown that in agreement with real data for the cities of New York and Chicago, that the rate of spread of the disease was proportional to the population density. In the present work, we added more realistic features, such as change of mobility within a city, which led to regions of the city with different densities, and the growth rate of the disease followed the trends of homogeneous high-density results. Another important consequence was that the mobility is smaller in high-density regions, which is a characteristic of Brownian diffusion, and this low mobility leads to high infection rates as the subjects tend to spend more time near each other.

Another major implementation in the present model was the interaction between two cities via interchange of travelers. We added on sick individual in one of the cities, and allowed two random travelers, one from each city to travel to the other city. The growth rate in the city with the initial traveler was the same as the results of the isolated city simulations. However, it was interesting to note in some simulations the disease did not spread to the other city. The probability to spread to the other city varied from 10% to 30%, depending on which city the first sick individual started from. To simulate more realistic travel patterns, we need to allow more individuals to travel to and from each of the cities. Nevertheless, the model does justify travel restrictions in cases of rapidly spreading lethal infections.

Finally, we implemented social distancing by means of a repulsive force. The results clearly show that the higher the level of social distancing compliance the lower the rate of infection, once again justifying this type of intervention to slow down the spread of future contagious diseases.

References

Acioli, P. H. (2020). Diffusion as a first model of spread of viral infection. *American Journal of Physics, 88*(8), 600–604. https://doi.org/10.1119/10.0001464

Andrews, A. (2021). Producing panic: An analysis of conspiracy theory rhetoric during the coronavirus pandemic of 2020. *Master's Theses*. University of Alabama in Huntsville, AL, United States of America.

Brooks, M. (2006). *World war Z*. The Crown Publishing Group, New York City.

Crichton, M. (1969). *The andromeda strain*. Knopf, New York City.

Dangerfield, C. E., Abrahams, I. D., Budd, C., Butchers, M., C. M., Champneys, A. R., ... & Wasley, D. (2023). Getting the most out of maths: How to coordinate mathematical modelling. *Journal of Theoretical Biology, 557*, 111332(1–12). https://doi. org/10.1016/j.jtbi.2022.111332

Defoe, D. (1772, 2003). *A journal of the plague year.* Penguin Books, London & New York.

Flynn, M. (1987, 2006). *Eifelheim.* Tor Books, New York City.

Herbert, F. (1982). *The White Plague.* G.P. Putnam's Sons, New York City.

Keller, M. S.-G. (2019). Ancient Yersinia pestis genomes from across Western Europe reveal early diversification during the first pandemic. *Proceedings of the National Academy of Sciences, 116*(25), 541–750. https://doi.org/10.1073/pnas.1820447116

Keyes, G. (2014). *Interstellar: The Official Movie Novelization.* Titan Books, London.

King, S. (1978). *The Stand.* Doubleday Publishing, New York City.

Littman, R. (2009). The plague of Athens: Epidemiology and paleopathology. *Mount Sinai Journal of Medicine: A Journal of Translational and Personalized Medicine, 76*(5), 456–467. https://doi.org/10.1002/msj.20137

Matheson, R. (1954). *I am legend.* Gold Medal Books, New York City.

Pais, C., Godano, M., Juarez, E., del Prado, A., Manresa, J., & Rufiner, H. (2023). City-scale model for COVID-19 epidemiology with mobility and social activities represented by a set of hidden Markov models. *Computers in Biology and Medicine, 160*, 106942. https://doi.org/10.1016/j.compbiomed.2023.106942

Sabbatani, S. F. S. (2009). La peste antonina e il declino dell'Impero Romano. Ruolo della guerra partica e della guerra marcomannica tra il 164 e il 182 d.c. nella diffusione del contagio [The Antonine Plague and the decline of the Roman Empire]. *Le Infezioni in Medicina, 17*(4), 261–75. Retrieved from https://pubmed.ncbi.nlm.nih. gov/20046111/

Sigler, S. (2008). *Infected.* The Crown Publishing Group, New York City.

Stewart, G. R. (1942). *Earth Abides.* Random House, Woodland Hills, CA.

Willis, C. (1992). *Doomsday Book.* Bantam Books/Random House, New York City.

Yang, H., Liu, H., & Li, G. (2023). A novel prediction model based on decomposition-integration and error correction for COVID-19 daily confirmed and death cases. *Computers in Biology and Medicine, 156*, 106674. https://doi.org/10.1016/j.compbiomed. 2023.106674

Conclusions and Implications

Marzenna Anna Weresa,
Christina Ciecierski and Lidia Filus

The improvement in society's health and well-being has been always an area of significant interest, but it gained particular importance after having been featured in the Social Development Goals of the United Nations (UN, 2015). The COVID-19 pandemic drew more attention to health and accelerated the process of the digitalization of the health system.

Digitalization of the health system is a heterogeneous issue covering a wide spectrum of health-related issues. The complexity of health digitalization is a result of the broad definition of a *health system*. The World Health Organization (WHO) defines health systems "as comprising all the organizations, institutions and resources that are devoted to producing health actions" (…), understood as "any effort, whether in personal health care, public health services or through intersectoral initiatives, whose primary purpose is to improve health." (WHO, 2000; 2022). The OECD also recognizes that improvements in people's health are regarded as the ultimate goal of health systems (OECD, 2021), and similar definitions are used by scholars (e.g., Arteaga, 2014). These definitions imply that digital health is about digitalization of all activities that are aimed at promoting, restoring, and/or maintaining health.

Since the outbreak of the COVID-19 pandemic, there has been a push toward the introduction of digital innovative solutions in the health system throughout the entire patient treatment process. These solutions range from internet- or phone-based health monitoring, through the use of digital solutions, in particular, artificial intelligence, in the diagnostics and treatment (Visconti & Morea, 2020; Taylor et al., 2022), to digital transformation of healthcare governance or digitalization of the pharmaceutical sector. Digitalization also occurs in the area of medical research and teaching, which may affect people's health in the long run. Thus, digital technologies have been shaping global health performance, and this was recognized by the WHO in the "Global Strategy on Digital Health 2020-2025" (WHO, 2021).

This book analyzes various digital health issues from an economic perspective. Having examined the nature of digital health innovation, the authors explain that the concept of digital health innovation is grounded in economics

DOI: 10.4324/9781032726557-12

of innovation, and at its core are radical and incremental innovations related to product and business processes. However, given the variety and diversity of areas where digital health innovation may occur, as well as its novelty and interdisciplinarity, this research field is still under development. The most intensive research on digital health innovation, as measured by the number of scientific publications, has been conducted in a few countries, with China and the US having the largest shares, followed by India, Canada, and the United Kingdom (UK). The research themes are clustered around the type of digital technology, mainly the health Internet of Things (IoT) and the use of big data and artificial intelligence.

When discussing digital health innovation, it is worth producing tangible, real-world examples. When providing just a few, radical innovations also need to be mentioned, such as the application of clinical genomics, pharmacogenomics, artificial intelligence algorithms, big data analytics in precision medicine across different types of patient data, and artificial intelligent optoelectronic skin or cloud-assisted Health IoT-enabled of electro-cardiogram monitoring.

Incremental digital health innovations include, for instance, electronic health records or IoT-based smart health devices (e.g. smart watches, health bands, and glucose monitoring devices) or iPad-compatible language translation applications employed in healthcare. Some of these new innovative solutions are quite complex, and they change not only performance of the overall health system but also, impact access to healthcare services. However, there are differences in digital readiness between the EU and the US with regard to resources and capacity, which may be significant when adopting digital health innovations. The analyses of this issue revealed some disparities between the EU and the US, the latter being more advanced in this respect. The European healthcare system is not homogeneous, with significant variations in the level of health digitalization among the EU member states. In particular, there is a gap in health digitalization between Western European countries and Central European countries (CEE).

Having compared the digital health readiness of EU and the US and concluding that the former has a weaker position than the latter, our analysis shifted focus to challenges posed by digital health development, with funding being one of them. A detailed study on the US experience based on the Markowitz model assumptions showed that investing in the digital health sector may be more attractive than investing in alternative assets (e.g., crude oil). Such investments can be regarded as a risk diversifier, and give the possibility of lower risk with a lower return for risk-averse investors compared to Bitcoin. The study on financing digital health also revealed that venture capital, business angels funds, or own capital, when combined with credit, are more promising methods for financing digital health than an initial public offering. Therefore, it seems that further development of venture capital markets can facilitate digital transformation of health systems.

In view of the disparities between Western Europe and the CEE countries that our studies revealed in regards to digital health readiness within the EU, the focus of our analyses shifted to Poland, the most populated EU member state in the CEE region. The key issues addressed through the detailed analyses of Poland's country case study include: a diagnosis of digitalization of Poland's healthcare system from a comparative perspective, followed by a closer look at telemedicine delivery in Poland and how it changed during and after the COVID pandemic.

Our studies show that Poland's performance in digital health is quite strong, matching and often surpassing the averages found in relatively more developed EU countries. Nonetheless, there are areas of digital health in which Poland lags including legislation, policy, compliance, and particularly, in the development of digital skills of the health sector workforce. There are also regional differences in health digitalization, in particular, a digital divide between Poland's urban versus rural areas. Further exploration of factors hampering remote consultations in Poland confirmed that one of the key barriers is a shortage of skill as well as difficulties in adapting to technological requirements among healthcare professionals and patients alike, in particular, patients who are older. Other barriers relate to technical difficulties, challenges in communications and security, regulations related to equipment and documentation, as well as an overall limited use of the digital patient-doctor relationship within certain healthcare fields, where face-to-face interactions appear to provide better emotional support (e.g., psychiatric care, palliative care).

In this context, the question arises about the future of digital health. A good example of an area where digitalization has already been of unquestionable value is medical research. This book also examines two scenarios of how big data and time series analysis are used to predict the outcomes of prescribed treatments for cancer as well as to forecast the spread of viruses. The former examines technologies that monitor clinical trials of oncological medications. Here, the diagnostics of medical parameters change over time and help to detect unwanted data patterns in order to make clinical trials of drugs more reliable. The latter shows how big data can be employed to predict outcomes of viral infections. Such research can be useful for policymakers in their design of new policy interventions which aim to limit the spread of viruses.

Summing up, this book contains diverse pieces of empirical evidence to show how digital technologies, and innovative digital solutions in particular, have been changing the landscape of health systems. A variety of real-life examples that derive from the US, the EU, and the case study of Poland relate to digital transformation and provide new insight into the digitalization of health systems.

Interconnectedness in the health system, which continues to intensify due to increasing digitalization, requires collaboration among all stakeholders, including patients, members of society as a whole, healthcare providers, payers (e.g., insurance companies), organizations financing the development and implementation of digital health solutions, public health institutions (e.g. WHO, universities, medical schools), policymakers, technology professionals, manufacturers of medical devices, pharmaceutical companies, etc.

The goal of the authors of this book is to share a wide spectrum of topics related to digital health, where each of focus areas studied here can be further explored. Our book only scratches the surface of these fascinating topics. There are plenty of avenues for future research which might center around health system players, in order to study the costs and benefits of health digitalization, as well as barriers to its continued advancement. A second approach might include a comparative analysis of countries and/or regions and their digital performance or alternatively, to focus on specific digital technologies and their applications across the health sector. The authors hope that the results of the research presented in this book will serve as an inspiration for further studies on digital health innovation.

References

Arteaga, O. (2014). Health systems. In A. C. Michalos (Ed.), *Encyclopedia of Quality of life and Well-being Research*. Springer, Dordrecht. https://doi.org/10.1007/978-94-007-0753-5_3390

OECD. (2021). *Health at a Glance 2021: OECD Indicators*. OECD Publishing, Paris, https://doi.org/10.1787/ae3016b9-en

Taylor, L., Giles, S., Howitt, S., Ryan, Z., Brooks, E., Radley, L., Thomson, A., Whitaker, E., Knight, F., Hill, C., Violato, M., Waite, P., Raymont, V., Yu, L.-M., Harris, V., Williams, N., & Creswell, C. (2022). A randomised controlled trial to compare clinical and cost-effectiveness of an online parent-led treatment for child anxiety problems with usual care in the context of COVID-19 delivered in Child and Adolescent Mental Health Services in the UK (Co-CAT): A study protocol for a randomised controlled trial. *Trials, 23*, 942. https://doi.org/10.1186/s13063-022-06833-5

UN. (2015). *Transforming Our World: The 2030 Agenda for Sustainable Development*. United Nations, Geneva. https://sdgs.un.org/2030agenda

Visconti, R. M., & Morea, D. (2020). Healthcare digitalization and pay-for-performance incentives in smart hospital project financing. *International Journal of Environmental Research and Public Health, 17*(7), 2318. https://doi.org/10.3390/ijerph17072318

WHO. (2000). *The World Health Report 2000. Health Systems: Improving Performance*. World Health Organization, Geneva. https://www.who.int/publications/i/item/924156198X

WHO. (2021). *Global Strategy on Digital Health 2020–2025*. World Health Organization, Geneva.

WHO. (2022). Health system performance assessment: A framework for policy analysis. *Health Policy Series, 57*. https://www.who.int/publications/i/item/9789240042476

Index

Note: **Bold** page numbers refer to tables and *italic* page numbers refer to figures.

Act on Medical Devices 72
Act on the Protection of Health
    Information and Medical
    Documentation 71
Act on the Protection of Personal
    Data 71
agent-based model 133
alternative assets 46–55, **47–52**, **54**, **55**
ambulatory care 90, 95
analyzed assets, correlation table for
    47–48
ARIMA model 117–119, 123
    CACRALB, subject 2 **121**
    LYM, subject 192 **126**
artificial intelligence 79, 149
    e-Health 67
    genomic analysis 14, 15
    healthcare 12
    Poland 72
augmented Dickey-Fuller (ADF) test
    117, 123
    CACRALB, subject 2 **121**
    LYM, subject 192 **126**
autocorrelation function (ACF) 117–119,
    123
    CACRALB, subject 2 *120*
    LYM, subject 192 *125*
autoregressive (AR) process 118

bankruptcy 37
bibliometric analysis 7, 15
    data 8
    results of 9–12, *10*, **11–12**
bibliometric methodology 9
big data 12, 14, 149
Bitcoin 43, 49, 149
    daily prices of *45*

descriptive statistics of logarithmic
    returns **50**
main statistics of logarithmic returns **54**
Black Death 132
blockchain 2, 15
Brent crude oil *46*, **50**
Brownian diffusion 146
Brownian motion 133, 134, 143

CACRALB, subject 2 118
    ACF and PACF plots for *120*
    ADF test results **121**
    ETS model summary **121**
    forecast accuracy **121**
    forecast comparison *122*
    outlier detection *124*
Canada 149
capabilities 18–29
capital 37–42, *38*, **40**; *see also* venture
    capital
case report form (CRF) 114
Centers for Disease Control and
    Prevention (CDC) 135–136
Central and Eastern Europe (CEE) 23,
    25, 26, 29, 149, 150
    comparative analysis 22
    healthy life expectancy 24
    physicians in 24
centralized monitoring (CM)
    defined 114
    frequency of on-site visits 114
    risk-based monitoring 114
    statistical methodology 115
central statistical monitoring (CSM)
    113–129
    principles of 114
    time series analysis 115

CeZ *see* e-Health Centre (CeZ)
China 11, 132, 149
Civil Status Registry 77
clinical data 114, 115, 117, 129
clinical time series 115
    diagnostics 117–126
    forecasting 118–126
clinical trials 2, 113–129, 150
    clinical time series diagnostics and
        forecasting 118–126
    correlation analysis 116–118
    data pre-processing 116
    discussion 126–129
    GSK plc 115
    introduction to 113–115
    laboratory variables **116**
    oncological medications 150
    risk-based monitoring 114
    study data tabulation model 116
    time series analysis 117–118
    variable selection 118
Code of Medical Ethics (CME), Article
    9 of 89
communication 21, 88
comparative analysis 18–29
comparative study 35–57
correlation analysis 116–118
correlation coefficients 46, **47–48**, 55, 56
correlation heatmap *119*
cost-effectiveness 77, 87
Council of Ministers of the Republic of
    Poland 72
COVID-19 pandemic 1, 7, 18, 19, 44,
    54, 89, 132, 133, 148, 150
    Chicago 133
    funding 36
    New York 133
    Parana City 133
    remote consultations 86
    social distancing 133
    teleconsultations 85–106
cross-border health data exchange 72
crude oil 43, 49
    daily prices of *46*
    main statistics of logarithmic
        returns **55**
cryptocurrency 56; *see also* Bitcoin
CSM *see* central statistical monitoring
    (CSM)
current health expenditure (CHE) 22

data collection 63–64
data pre-processing 116
data research 63–64

diffusion constant 134–136
    exponential growth rate **137**, **138**
    with population density 137, 140
    two-diffusion constant simulation
        cell *141*
diffusion model 143–146
Digital Competence Development
    Programme 72
Digital Decade policy program 102
digital economy 1
Digital Economy and Society Index
    (DESI) 102
digital health 1, 2, 19
    financing 37–42, *38*, **40**
    how to analyze the state of 64
    importance 63–64
    inequalities 20
    IPO 35–57
    maturity assessment models
        comparison 64, **65**
    maturity overview for Poland *80*
    start-ups 41
    stocks 35, 43, 46, 49, 52, 53, 56
    venture capital 36, 37–42, *38*, **40**
    WHO reports 8
Digital Health Business &
    Technology 36
digital health financing 35–37, 56, 149
Digital Health Index, in Poland 66
    Infrastructure 75–76, **76**
    introduction to 63–64
    Leadership & Governance 67–68, **69**
    Legislation, Policy, &
        Compliance 70–72, **73**
    methodology 64–66
    Services & Applications 76–78,
        78–79
    Standards & Interoperability 73–75,
        75
    Strategy & Investment 68–70, **71**
    Workforce 72–73, **74**
digital health innovation 2, 7–16, 18, 20,
    148, 149, 151
    bibliometric analysis 9–12, *10*, **11–12**
    bibliometric methodology 9
    incremental 149
    introduction to 7
    main findings from the literature
        review 13–15, **14**
    methodology and data **8**, 8–9
    thematic and network analysis
        12–13, *13*
Digital Health Profile (DHP) 64, 81
digital health transformation, US 35–57

factors influencing opportunities
37–42, *38*, **40**
final findings and limitations 56–57
general equity market and alternative
assets 46–55, **47–52**, **54**, **55**
introduction to 35–36
literature overview 36–37
methodology *43*, 43–44, *45*, *46*
digital innovations 1, 2, 13, 22
COVID-19 pandemic 7, 148
in health 7, 14, **14**, 15
healthcare industry 20
OECD/Eurostat 14
digitalization 1, 18, 19, 21, 22, 148, 150
Central and Eastern European
countries 29
health 1, 149, 151
healthcare 2, 21, 23, 29, **29**
medical research and teaching 148
Poland's healthcare system 150
society 24, 26
digital readiness, in healthcare 18–29
data and methods 22
introduction to 18–19
literature review 19–22
results **23**, 23–26, *25*, *27*, *28*
digital technology 12, *13*, 19, 21
digital transformation 1, 2, 20, 21, 36,
80, 148–150
diversity 68, 149
domestic private health expenditure
(PVT-D) 22, *27*

Ebola 132, 133
e-counselling 21
effectiveness 20
of remote consultations 87
e-government services 102
Egypt 132
e-health/e-Health 20, 36, 72
artificial intelligence 67
Ministry of Health 67
research 16
US funding 36
e-Health Centre (CeZ) 68, 76, 77, 79
analytical and architectural
environment 74
architectural repository 73, 74, 81
artificial intelligence 67
data model standardization 74
electronic cross-border patient card
solutions 72, **73**
interop e-government systems 74
operations 70

e-Health Centre Development Strategy
75, 78
e-Health Centre Strategy (2023–2027)
67, 70
e-Health Development Programme 67,
68, 70, 71, 75
electronic health records 15; *see also*
e-health/e-Health
electronic medical records (EMR) 22,
24, 29
electronic records 21
electronic registries 21
Enterprise Architect (EA) 74
entrepreneurs 38, 39, 57
epidemics 133, 141, 142, 144, 145
equality 68
equity 37, 41, 42, 70
ETS model 117–119, 123
CACRALB, subject 2 **121**
LYM, subject 192 **126**
European Commission 19
European Strategic Plan (2019–2024) 19
European Union (EU) 1, 72, 80, 149
AI use, in healthcare services 72
comparative analysis of 18–29
Digital Economy and Society Index
102
digital readiness 149, 150
General Data Protection Regulation
70, 80
5G technology 102
European Union (EU-15) 22, 24, 25
electronic medical records 24
healthy life expectancy 24

face-to-face consultations 86, 87,
104–106
financial incentives 89
financing 2, 89, 96
debt 42
digital health 36, 56, 149
healthcare 25
initial public offering 37–42
organizations 150
private 35
public market 57
teleconsultations 100
venture capital 37
5G technology 102
forecast accuracy, CACRALB, subject
2 **121**
forecast comparison
CACRALB, subject 2 *122*
LYM, subject 192 *127*

fraud detection 115
funding 35–57, 68

Gaussian distribution 134
General Data Protection Regulation
    (GDPR) 70, 80
general equity market 46–55, **47–52,
    54, 55**
general government health
    expenditure *25*
generalized diffusion model 132–146
    discussion 143–146
    introduction to 132–133
    methods 133–134
    results 134–142, *135–142*, **137, 138**
general practitioners, teleconsultations
    89, 90
    by age groups **92**
    by month *91*
    voivodeship *92*
genomic analysis 14, 15
Global Digital Health Index (GDHI) 66
Global Strategy on Digital Health (2020–
    2025) 148
Great Plague of London 132
GSK plc 115, 129

HALE *see* healthy life expectancy
    (HALE)
health 1, 7, 18, 63, 72, 77, 93, 95, 105,
    148, 149; *see also* digital health
    crises, response to 64
    data transmission 15
    equity 64
    information networks 21
    long-term viability 19
healthcare 7, 63–64, 72, 77, 81, 85–87,
    90, 104
    access to 19, 20, 63
    artificial intelligence 12, 67
    availability 19, 21
    big data 12
    digital readiness in 18–29
    digital transformation in 20
    Europe, challenges 19
    expenditure 25
    financial incentives 89
    financing 25
    iPad-compatible language translation
        apps in 15
    public and private expenditure 18
    reform 93
    in Uruguay 22

healthcare providers 18, 21, 44, 63,
    85–90, 96, 101, 104, 150
    consultation details 104
    reimbursement products 102
Health Internet of Things (HIoT) 12
healthy life expectancy (HALE) 22, 24,
    25, 25, *27*
human rights 68

income-related inequality 22
India 15, 132, 149
Industry 4.0 1 20
inequality 19, 68
    digital health 20
    income-related 22
    pro-rich 22
Infectious Dynamics of Pandemic
    (IDP) 133
information and communication
    technologies (ICT) 68, 73, 88
information asymmetry 38, 42
Infrastructure category, in Polish digital
    health 75–76, **76**
initial public offering (IPO) 35–57
    average return of 41
    strengths and weaknesses of 37–42,
        38, **40**
    withdrawing funds 41
innovation, digital health *see* digital
    health innovation
innovative interventions 19
Integrated Analytical Model 78, 81
interconnectedness 150
Internet 21, 22, 26, *27*, *28*
Internet of Things (IoT) 15, 149
Internet Patient Account (IKP) 77
inverse care law 19
IPO *see* initial public offering (IPO)

Kensho index *see* S&P Kensho index

laws safeguarding 80
Leadership & Governance category, in
    Polish digital health 67–68, **69**
Legislation, Policy, & Compliance
    category, in Polish digital health
    70–72, **73**
liquidity 41, 42
logarithmic returns
    Bitcoin **50, 54**
    Brent crude oil **50**
    crude oil **55**
    S&P 500 TR Index **48, 49, 51, 52**

long-term care (LTC) 99, *100*
LYM, subject 192 123
  ACF and PACF plots for *125*
  ADF test results **126**
  ARIMA model summary **126**
  ETS model summary **126**
  forecast comparison *127*
  forecast summary **126**
  outlier detection *128*

macroeconomic data 18, 22
mapping the research field 7–16
market stabilization 41
Markowitz theory 51, 53, 56, 149
measles 132
Medicaid 23
medical appointment 22
medical care 21–22
Medicare 23
Ministry of Digital Affairs 77
Ministry of Health 67, 71, 79
mixed-method research 90
mobility 133, 143, 144, 146
moving average (MA) process 118

NASDAQ 44
National Broadband Plan 102
National Health Fund (NFZ) 88, 96, 103
National Health Programme 68
National Plan for Reconstruction and
  Increasing Resilience 68
National Recovery Plan (KPO) 76
nature of digital health innovation 7–16
network analysis 12–13
Network Readiness Index (NRI) score 75
New York Stock Exchange 44
non-compliance 89

Office for Personal Data Protection
  (UODO) 70
The Open Group Architecture
  Framework (TOGAF) 74
outlier detection
  CACRALB, subject 2 *124*
  LYM, subject 192 *128*
outpatient specialist care,
  teleconsultations 93
  by month *94*
  voivodeship *94*

palliative-hospice care 99, **101**
partial autocorrelation function (PACF)
  117, 118

CACRALB, subject 2 *120*
  LYM, subject 192 *125*
patient-doctor contact 95
patient engagement 63
Pearson correlation coefficient 44, 46,
  116
per capita healthcare expenditure 23, 28
physical examination 87, 104
plague of Athens 132
Plague of Cyprian 132
Plague of Justinian 132
Poland 2, 150
  Act on the Protection of Personal
    Data 71
  AI, development policy 72
  Digital Health Index 63–81
  digital health maturity overview *80*
  Digital Health Profile 64
  doctors per capita 26, *27*
  domestic government spending on
    healthcare 25
  e-Health Centre Strategy
    (2023–2027) 70
  e-Health development 75
  General Data Protection Regulation 70
  5G technology 102
  infrastructure development 75
  Internet infrastructure 102
  Network Readiness Index 75, 81
  teleconsultations in 85–106
  treatment capacity 19
Polish Digital Transformation Strategy
  102
Polish e-prescriptions 72
Polish healthcare system 88–90
population density 134, 135, *135*, *136*
  Chicago 140, *142*
  diffusion constant with 137, 140
  NYC 140, *142*
  two-diffusion constant simulation cell
    139, *140*
portable devices 21
Primary Healthcare Facility (POZ) 89
private financing 35
private healthcare expenditure 25
professional ethics 89
pro-rich inequality 22
psychiatric care services 96
  for adults **96**
  for voivodeship *97*
  for youth and children **97**
public company 41–42
public health 63–64

quality of care 63

Rapid Assistance in Modelling the
    Pandemic (RAMP) 133
RBQM *see* risk-based quality
    management (RBQM)
remote consultations
    benefits of 85
    clinical outcomes 87
    concept of 85
    cost-effectiveness 87
    COVID-19 pandemic 86
    effectiveness of 87
    global pandemic 86
    healthcare delivery 86
    legal framework, Polish healthcare
        system 88–90
    physical interaction, lack of 88
    popularity and widespread use 88
    reduce waiting times 86
remote monitoring 15, 44
returns 44; *see also* logarithmic returns
risk-based monitoring (RBM) 114
risk-based quality management
    (RBQM) 114
Rock Health 36
R software 8
Russia-Ukraine war 44

Safavi, K. C. 36
SARS 132
SDTM *see* study data tabulation model
    (SDTM)
secondary research 35
Services & Applications category, in
    Polish digital health 76–78, **78–79**
SES model 118
Shore, J. H. 87
short-term immunity 134
skewness 44, 49, 53
smallpox 132
SNOMED clinical terminology 75
social distancing 85, 133, 146
societal change 93
source data review (SDR) 113
source data verification (SDV) 113
source documentation 113
Spanish flu 132
S&P Kensho index 38, 43, 44, 46, 53, 56
    alternative assets and 50
    average return 46
    remote healthcare services 44
    skewness 53
    stock market quotations *43*

S&P 500 Total Return index 43, 44
    descriptive statistics of logarithmic
        returns **48**, **49**
    kurtosis 48
    main statistics of logarithmic
        returns **51**
    stock market quotations of *45*
standard deviations 44, 49, 53, 56
Standards & Interoperability category, in
    Polish digital health 73–75, **75**
start-ups 37, 41
statistical simulations 134, 144
stock market 36, 41, 44, 56
    crash 37
    equity 37
    S&P Kensho index *43*
    S&P 500 Total Return index *45*
    US 42
Strategic Framework for Health Care in
    Poland 68
Strategy & Investment category, in
    Polish digital health 68–70, **71**
study data tabulation model (SDTM) 116
Sustainable Development Goals
    (SDG) 29

telecardiology 88
telecommunications tools 85
teleconsultations 85–106; *see also*
    remote consultations
    AOS services *94*
    discussion 101–105
    epidemiological situation 98
    general practitioners *91–92*, **92**
    introduction to 85–86
    long-term care services *99*
    methods 90
    palliative and hospice care **101**
    psychiatric care services **96**, **97**,
        97, 98
    remote consultations 88–90
    results 90–101
    state of the art 86–88
telegeriatrics 88
telehealth 85, 86
    guidelines and policies 88
    inequities 88
    technical issues 88
telemedicine 15, 19, 21, 79, 85, 86, 103
    cost savings 87
    heart failure 87
    patient satisfaction 87
telemonitoring 15
telepsychiatry 105

thematic analysis 12–13
time series analysis (TSA) 113–129
    clinical time series diagnostics
        117–118
    clinical time series forecasting 118
    multivariate 129
Total Return Index 44; *see also* S&P 500
    Total Return index
traditional face-to-face
    consultations 87
treasury bills 41
treasury securities 41
TSA *see* time series analysis (TSA)
two-diffusion constant simulation cell
    139–141

United Nations Agenda (2030) 1
United States (US) 11, 149
    Centers for Disease Control and
        Prevention 135–136
    comparative analysis of 18–29
    digital health transformation 35–57
    digital readiness 149
    Ebola outbreak 133
    e-health funding 36
    electronic medical records 24, 29
    healthcare financing 26
    Medicaid 23
    Medicare 23
    physicians in 24

plague 132
telehealth visits 86
univariate statistical analysis 114
Universal Health Coverage (UHC) 29,
    66, 70, 80

variable selection 118
venture capital 35–57
    capital flows 38, *38*
    digital health (2011–2023) **40**
    fundings 35
    investments 36
    investors 36
    strengths and weaknesses of 37–42,
        38, **40**
venture capitalists 39, 41, 56
viral spread 132–146
virtual appointments 86
Virtual Forum for Knowledge Exchange
    in Mathematical Sciences (V-KEMS)
    133

Workforce category, in Polish digital
    health 72–73, **74**
World Health Organization (WHO) 29
    digital health 8
    Global Digital Health Strategy 66
    Global Strategy on Digital Health
        (2020–2025) 148
    health systems 148

Milton Keynes UK
Ingram Content Group UK Ltd.
UKHW031137141024
449569UK00006B/123